D1376125

Confuse and Conceal

PCTs Library Oldham & Tameside

BN05757

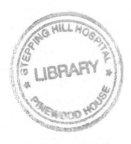

STEPPING HILL HOSPITAL
LIBRARY
PINEWOOD HOUSE

CONFUSE & CONCEAL
THE NHS AND INDEPENDENT
SECTOR TREATMENT CENTRES

Stewart Player and Colin Leys

MERLIN PRESS

© Stewart Player & Colin Leys, 2008

First published 2008 by The Merlin Press Ltd.
96 Monnow Street
Monmouth
NP25 3EQ
Wales

www.merlinpress.co.uk

ISBN 9780850366099

Stewart Player and Colin Leys have asserted their right to be
identified as the authors of this work under the Copyright,
Designs and Patents Act 1988

British Library Cataloguing in Publication Data
is available from the British Library

All rights reserved. No part of this publication may be
reproduced, stored in a retrieval system, or transmitted,
in any form or by any means, electronic, mechanical,
photocopying, recording or otherwise, without the
prior permission of the publisher.

Printed in the EU by L.P.P.S. Ltd. NN8 3PJ

Contents

List of Acronyms

ACAD	Ambulatory Care and Diagnostic Centre
AvMA	Action Against Medical Accidents, formerly Association of Victims of Medical Accidents
BMA	British Medical Association
BMJ	British Medical Journal
BOA	British Orthopaedic Association
CASS	Community Assessment Support Spoke
CATS	Clinical Assessment and Treatment Service
CNST	Clinical Negligence Scheme for Trusts
DGH	District General Hospital
DH	Department of Health
ECN	Extended Choice Network
ENT	Ear Nose and Throat
FCE	Finished Consultant Episode
FFS	Fee for Service
FOI	Freedom of Information
GP	General Practitioner, or General Practice
ICATS	Integrated Clinical Assessment and Treatment Service
ISCB	Independent Sector Commissioning Board
ISTC	Independent Sector Treatment Centre
KPI	Key Performance Indicator
MSA	Market Sustainability Analysis
NCHOD	National Centre for Health Outcomes Development
NCSC	National Care Standards Commission
NHSLA	National Health Service Litigation Authority
NHS TC	NHS Treatment Centre
NIT	National Implementation Team
NLN	National Leadership Network for Health and Social Care
OECD	Organization for Economic Cooperation and Development
PCT	Primary Care Trust
PSC	Public Sector Comparator
SHA	Strategic Health Authority
VFM	Value for Money

Foreword by Dr Wendy Savage

This book should be read by all those who understand and cherish the principles on which the National Health Service (NHS) was founded. It should also be compulsory reading for all Members of Parliament, civil servants and non-executive members of Boards of Primary Care Trusts and Hospital Trusts and Strategic Health Authorities. As the 60th anniversary of the foundation of the first freely available health service approaches, and 10 years after we greeted the election of a Labour government with relief, the threat to the NHS as we know it is serious, and if we as a nation do not act vigorously now, will lead to irreversible damage.

Stewart Player and Colin Leys have managed to get behind the government spin about choice and the 'Patient led NHS'. The contents of the Department of Health's frequent press releases are usually reported accurately by the media but without any critical analysis or in-depth scrutiny. Using quotes from Department of Health (DH) policy documents and evidence given to the House of Commons Health Committee, which looked at ISTCs in 2006, supplemented by Freedom of Information requests, the authors make a convincing case for a conspiracy to change the NHS irrevocably. The government has stated that its aim is to create a health care market and former Health Secretary Patricia Hewitt said that there was to be no limit to the involvement of the private sector in this market.

In the first chapter they examine the setting up of the so-called 'Independent Sector Treatment Centres' (ISTCs) and the role of the little-known Commercial Directorate, and attempt to estimate how much work the first wave ISTCs have performed. They suggest that the reduction in the number of second wave ISTCs was not, as some commentators assumed, a sign that the government was having second thoughts about NHS reform: it was because they had achieved its objective of introducing the private sector into the NHS. The programme could now move on to the next phase, of changing the private health care sector and extending its role within the NHS. This theme is developed more in chapter 3. The detailed and comprehensive collection of statistics is invaluable in understanding what is happening within the NHS under the cloak of wordy and turgid policy documents and rhetoric about patient choice embodied in 'Creating a patient-led NHS ' March 2005 and 'Commissioning a patient-led NHS' July 2005.

Their analysis, in the second chapter, of the House of Commons' Health Committee's investigation into ISTCs in 2006 is illuminating but depressing. It shows clearly how the Committee failed on many counts to scrutinise effectively the ISTC programme. Despite one member describing the programme as 'an evidence-free zone' they did not confront the DH when it refused to give details of cost because of 'commercial confidentiality'. How can a government department, spending taxpayers' money, be allowed to do this by the Parliamentary Committee which should be overseeing the actions of the government on behalf of the citizens who have elected them to office? The Committee did not pursue important leads such as that given by Professor John Appleby about the creation of a health care market. It accepted the view of the DH, which considered the programme was working well, even though the Department had failed to set up a proper system for monitoring the outcomes of ISTCs' clinical work and so had no hard data to support this view. The evidence collected by the British Orthopaedic Association appears to contradict the government's complacent assessment of how effective the ISTCs have proved to be, but was discounted by the Committee. The evidence that showed that the need for ISTCs was not decided locally but imposed from the centre was apparently accepted by the Committee but it did not pursue the matter, despite the bullying tactics that were clearly used to ensure that PCT members complied with the Department's plans. In short, in spite of considerable scepticism over many of the DH claims, the Committee failed to protect the public by exposing the nature of the government's programme and this failure has profound implications for the way our democracy functions.

The third chapter gives a detailed account of the mechanisms employed in setting up a health care market and reports on the Extended Choice Network launched in May 2006, designed to keep the private sector engaged in the programme. A considerable number of private hospitals are now included in the Choose and Book programme so that by 2008 patients would have increased choice at a price the DH was prepared to sanction. The use of NHS staff to work in ISTCs, the setting-up of chambers of doctors who will contract their services, often on a fee per service basis, and bonuses for individual doctors and nurses, are being introduced without public knowledge or scrutiny, despite the known risks of this type of approach. Increasingly, doctors and nurses will no longer be employed by the NHS and the integrated service that has been built up over 60 years will be fragmented and ultimately destroyed. Already health policymakers are predicting medical unemployment even though the UK still has fewer doctors per head of population than the majority of OECD countries.

Today, 1st January 2008, I read Gordon Brown's message to NHS staff on the DH website. He thanks them for their dedication but does not mention the changes discussed in this book although referring to the achievements over the last 10 years. He says:

> For sixty years now Britain has shown the way to health care not as a privilege to be paid for but as a fundamental human right. The NHS remains our priority not just because it has been fundamental to our past, but because a renewed NHS will be even more important to our future and that of our children.

He suggests we need a NHS constitution and a continuation of the reform programme to meet the challenges of the 21st century but how can the ideals of the NHS persist in the face of the emphasis on marketisation? Those who have seen Sicko, Michael Moore's film about the US health care system, or who know about the 47 million uninsured, and the glaring inequalities in the USA, which has poorer health outcomes nationally than poor counties like Cuba and almost all of Europe, know this is not the way for the UK to go. This book is not an easy read to be skimmed over in an hour or so but a serious account which clearly sets out, with detailed references and timetables, what is happening to our NHS, using taxpayers' money to confuse and conceal what is being done. As Aneurin Bevan MP said of the NHS, *'It will survive as long as there are folk left with the faith to fight for it'*. It is time for the public to wake up to what is happening to the NHS and join together to resist this transformation by all means possible.

Dr Wendy Savage MBBCh MSc HonDSc FRCOG, Honorary Professor at Middlesex University School of Health and Social Policy, Chair of Keep Our NHS Public Steering Group. The Keep Our NHS Public website address is: www.keepournhspublic.com

Preface

This book began life as a report intended primarily for readers involved in making or analysing health policy, but it turned out to raise issues that must concern everyone who cares about the future of the NHS or, indeed, the democratic process itself. The ISTC programme is a key part of a policy to convert the NHS into a healthcare market. It is being pushed ahead, with ministerial support, by a combination of bureaucratic and business actors, and some clinicians, as far as possible out of public view.

There is a very striking difference between what is said within the 'policy community' of people who have devised the policy, or are privy to it and are carrying it out, and what is reported in the national media. The house journals of the private healthcare industry regularly report policy developments which are publicly divulged much later, if at all, in the national press, and often seem not to be fully conveyed to MPs. On the other hand information published by the Department of Health on the marketisation programme tends to be at once technical and imprecise – the researcher never seems to get the same answer twice – and information reported in the national press is often contradictory and confusing. Before the 2005 election Tony Blair's policy advisers had a phrase for testing manifesto ideas for public service reform – 'further, faster, bigger, madder'. This sentiment was understood and appreciated by the market, but always downplayed by ministers in public. The situation does not seem to have changed much under Gordon Brown. When the new government took office corporate health care providers were quickly reassured by the Director General of the Department of Health's Commercial Directorate that the government was still working 'unceasingly' to create a 'level playing field' for independent providers to compete with the NHS. There seems to be every reason to believe him.

Getting at the facts about the ISTC programme (which one MP described, with some justice, as 'an evidence-free policy zone') has not been easy, and we have needed and used help and advice from many people. Given the controversial nature of the topic it seems wisest not to thank them by name, though we must make an exception for Julian Tudor Hart who, without intending to, kindly supplied us with our title. But the others know who they are, and they have our very sincere thanks.

Stewart Player
Colin Leys
December 2007

Introduction

The Independent Sector Treatment Centre (ISTC) programme has been presented to Parliament and the public as primarily about using private healthcare companies (the 'independent sector') to shorten waiting times for elective surgery and diagnostic tests, and to introduce greater choice. In reality it is a critical step towards the conversion of the NHS into a market in which for-profit providers will compete with NHS providers. Private companies are already providing a small but growing share of NHS primary care, through 'walk-in centres', 'out of hours' services and (in some areas) the provision of complete General Practices. ISTCs represent the first step in bringing private companies into the regular provision of NHS secondary care.

The government has declared that there is no upper limit to the proportion of the NHS budget that will in future be spent on private provision,[1] and NHS trusts are already cutting services as patient income is diverted to private providers. As provision by private companies expands, provision by NHS trusts will be increasingly slimmed down and clinical personnel will increasingly be employed by the private sector. ISTCs, and over 150 private hospitals that are now said to be ready to compete with NHS trusts at NHS rates,[2] are already having this effect. In addition, some of the ISTCs due to open in the second phase of the programme are 'referral centres' known as Clinical Assessment and Treatment Services centres, or CATS, again run by private companies, through which GPs' referrals for specialist care will be routed. Simultaneously other private companies, drawn from an approved list of fourteen, are being contracted to take over commissioning from PCTs.[3] As competition intensifies, the deciding factor in who gets what treatment will increasingly be profitability rather than health need.

The establishment of ISTCs and CATS as permanent features of the NHS represents a critical moment in the dissolution of the NHS as an integrated nation-wide health service in England. But because this is not a popular aim it is being pushed through without serious parliamentary debate. Public information about ISTCs is kept to a minimum. Such data as are released are very limited and of questionable quality. The only detailed official enquiry, conducted in 2006 by the House of Commons Health Select Committee, failed to confront evidence which pointed to the real aim of the ISTC programme. The Committee also failed to register a significant protest when Department of Health (DH) representatives appearing before it deliberately obfuscated key issues, and in particular refused to give the Committee financial information needed for evaluating the ISTC programme effectively in terms of the goals officially claimed for it.[4]

This book aims to present and analyse what is known about ISTCs in three distinct steps. First, in Chapter 1, we describe the genesis of the programme, its implementation, and its general characteristics.

Second, in Chapter 2, we review the House of Commons Health Select Committee's enquiry. Following the line taken by the Committee, we take the official aims of the programme one by one and try to assess the evidence on the extent to which they have been met. In each case we look first at the evidence given to the Committee, and then comment on the Committee's handling of it. We conclude that the Committee allowed itself to take the government's presentation of the aims of the ISTC programme at face value, and neglected to consider its true ulterior aim. As a result its report contained several significant inconsistencies. It also tended to downplay evidence that questioned the government's claims, and failed to comment forcefully on matters that did give it cause for concern. We also look briefly at the Healthcare Commission's report on the quality of care provided by ISTCs, which revealed some similar shortcomings. Neither body effectively held the government to account.

Finally, in Chapter 3, we look at some of the evidence that shows how the ISTC programme fits into the government's longer-term strategy for creating a fully market-driven healthcare system, focusing on elements in the strategy that are particularly significant for understanding the role of ISTCs.

Notes

1   John Carvel, 'Hewitt rules out limiting size of private sector role in NHS', *Guardian,* September 20, 2006.

2   Freedom of Information response from the Department of Health, DE00000228102, 13 August 2007.

3   'Backing for private sector's NHS role', *Financial Times* 5 October 2007.

4   House of Commons Health Committee, *Independent Sector Treatment Centres,* Fourth Report of Session 2005-06 (hereafter HC Report), Vol I, p. 37, para. 103.

CHAPTER 1: THE ISTC PROGRAMME – ITS HISTORY AND CHARACTERISTICS

Treatment centres in general

The Labour Government's *NHS Plan* of July 2000 announced a major programme of investment and reform of the National Health Service. A key element in the *Plan* was the reduction in waiting times for elective treatment.[1] Unless separate resources of staff and facilities are provided for non-emergency care there is always a tendency for planned, clinical procedures such as knee and hip replacements to be postponed to allow emergency cases to be dealt with. To overcome this, starting in 1999, NHS Treatment Centres were established, formalizing a practice already adopted in some NHS hospitals. Sixteen NHS Treatment Centres were already in existence by April 2002, when the government announced a new programme of dedicated and separate centres, to perform a high volume of relatively straightforward elective procedures in a predictable flow, 'to help meet NHS waiting time reductions and provide more rapid, convenient and improved outpatient and diagnostic services in the community…diversify service provision and, once again, relieve pressure on mainstream NHS hospitals'.[2] These centres were seen as central to achieving the government's aim of ensuring that by 2008 no patient should wait longer than 18 weeks from the time of GP referral to receiving a needed elective treatment. By January 2007 there were 43 NHS treatment centres, which in 2005-2006 had provided 186,355 elective procedures.[3]

The additional investment promised in the *NHS Plan*, however, was also predicated upon a more constructive engagement between the NHS and the private sector, in order to 'harness the capacity of private and voluntary providers to treat more NHS patients'.[4] This included inviting private providers to establish treatment centres too. By April 2002 a White Paper, *Delivering the NHS Plan: next steps on investment, next steps on reform*, reported that 'the first arrangements for the private sector to provide treatment centres are under negotiation', the 'first clinical teams having [already] been brought in from abroad in order to boost NHS surgical capacity'.[5]

A DH prospectus of June 2002 explicitly described this programme as involving 'the creation of a new sector in health care provision in England'. The new sector would be:

> (i) additional to existing publicly owned NHS provision; (ii) radically different from traditional usage of the private sector, not least in that the NHS will be the core business of units in this sector; and (iii) distinctive from other attempts to use spare capacity, such as treatment abroad, in that the services will be provided in this country and that these units will be managed and operated as independent sector units.[6]

Most later pronouncements, however, including the evidence given by the Department of Health to the Health Committee in 2006, did not stress this aim.

The defining characteristics of the ISTC programme were to be:

- The highest levels of quality heath care productivity: these units will offer trail-blazing levels of clinically effective, efficient, integrated, patient-centred care pathways;
- Real increases in the number of medical professionals working in England: the medical staff in these units will be from overseas, or otherwise additional to the existing NHS workforce; and
- High value for money: the productivity levels of such units will be such that they can offer services at competitive unit costs.[7]

Further aims were spelled out in a policy paper of December 2002 devoted specifically to ISTCs (*Growing Capacity: Independent Sector Diagnosis and Treatment* Centres), including the delivery of value for money through 'robust, competitive tendering'; to be efficient, effective and fast; and to have a focus on outputs (expressed in finished clinical activity) to provide incentives for the outcomes the NHS needed (such as additional activity and productivity improvements).[8] Pricing would eventually be based on the national tariff.

Procurement would take two different forms: (i) national procurement, led by a national implementation manager, to 'address a number of capacity gaps through the provision of multiple DTC [Diagnostic and Treatment Centre] units, and some specific schemes; (ii) local procurement for specific schemes 'where the procurement [would] be led by the project itself with enabling from a central team in the DH (providing advice and support on commercial and legal issues)'.[9]*

Independent Sector Treatment Centres, Wave 1

The Wave 1 ISTC programme was 'expected to provide an average of over 170,000 Finished Consultant Episodes (FCEs) a year over five years, and represent[ed] an investment of approximately £1.6 billion'.[10] The first ISTC contracts were signed in September 2003, and the first centre, owned by the Birkdale Clinic, opened in Daventry, Northamptonshire, the following month. Table 1 shows the companies involved, the centres they own, and the types and total numbers of procedures contracted for.

*'DTC' was the original term used; this has now been replaced with ISTC. East Berkshire PCT's Full Business Case from March 2004 provides a useful summary: 'The ISTC programme was initiated after a capacity review of NHS provision in the UK was completed in 2002. This review found that there were gaps in provision up and down the nation, which needed to be addressed. Following the capacity review some health economies, ("Gaps"), entered the programme on their own and are known as Local Schemes. Other Gaps were clustered together to form what are known as a Chain Schemes. The Spine Chain is the largest of all the chains within the programme and is comprised of 11 Gaps that span the length of the country, from Cornwall up to Newcastle. The East Berkshire Gap is part of the Spine Chain, which is also known as "GC4"'.

Table 1. Wave 1 of the ISTC programme by original provider, project, and number of procedures over the contract period of 5 years:

PROVIDER	PROJECTS	TYPES OF PROCEDURE PROVIDED	NUMBER OF PROCEDURES
NETCARE	Ophthalmic Spine Chain (Northumberland, Cumbria, Lancashire, Cheshire, Se London, Surrey, Hampshire, Sw Peninsula); Greater Manchester.	Ophthalmology	89,600
CAPIO	East Corwall; E Lincs; W Lincs; Horton; Neynl; Southampton; Northumberland; Thames Valley 3500; Gc4 West Surrey	Ophthalmology; General Surgery; Orthopaedics; Gastroenterology; Urology; Gynaecology; Colonoscopies; Trauma; Minor Skin; Upper Scopes; Dermatology; Varicose Veins; Hernias; Minor Surgery	93,441
MERCURY	Brighton; Wycombe; Medway; Portsmouth; Havant	Orthopaedics; General Surgery; Ent; Oral Surgery; Gastroenterology; Urology; Diagnostics	498,151
NATIONS HEALTHCARE	Nottingham; Bradford; Burton	Ophthalmology; Orthopaedics; Ent; Gynaecology; General Surgery; Gastroenterology; Plastics; Urology; Oral Surgery; Ultrasounds; Rheumatology	276,680
PARTNERSHIP HEALTH GROUP	Maidstone; Outer Ne London; Plymouth	Ophthalmology; Orthopaedics; Ent; Oral Surgery; General Surgery; Urology; Diagnostics	128,144
INTERHEALTH	Kidderminster; Cheshire & Merseyside;	Orthopaedics	33,817
CLINICENTA	Lister Surgi Centre; Hemel Hempstead	Ophthalmology; Ent; Paediatrics; Endoscopies; Urology; Gynaecology;	158,845
UK SPECIALIST HOSPITALS	Shepton Mallet	Ophthalmology; Orthopaedics; General Surgery; Endoscopies	56,242
BIRKDALE CLINIC	Daventry	Ophthalmology; Orthopaedics; Plastics; Oral Surgery; Endoscopies	5,959
TOTAL NUMBER OF PROCEDURES OVER FIVE YEARS			1,310,879

Source: Department of Health's submission to the Health Committee, HC Report Vol. II, Ev.1, pps 2-37

Table 2. Wave 1: Procedures contracted for by specialty:

PROCEDURES	NUMBER OF PROCEDURES CONTRACTED FOR UNDER WAVE 1
GENERAL SURGERY	299,000
ORTHOPAEDIC AND SPINAL	293,000
OPHTHALMOLOGY	122,000
UROLOGY	73,000
ENT	50,000
GYNAECOLOGY	38,000
CARDIOTHORACIC	4,000
TOTAL NUMBER OF PROCEDURES	879,000*

Source: Freedom of Information Request DE00000189579; Received 27 March 2007.
*The difference between the totals in the two tables remains to be accounted for. An FOI request was pending in December 2007.

Phase 1 ISTC Contracts

It is important to stress that no ISTC contracts are available for inspection by Parliament or the public. The disposal of the £5.6 billion committed to Wave 1 and Phase 2 is treated as commercially confidential. What is known is only how the contracts were procured, and their general nature, as outlined below.* Some further insight can be gleaned from some of the business cases prepared prior to the making of contracts, and from what the Department of Health told the Health Committee about how value for money was judged, both of which are discussed in Chapter 2.

a) Central procurement

ISTC contracts are between the private providers and Primary Care Trusts (PCTs), which pay for them out of the funds allocated to them by the Strategic Health Authorities (SHAs). Deciding where ISTCs should be located, however, and how many procedures each should be contracted to undertake, was the responsibility of the Department of Health. Most ISTCs belong to 'chains', owned by a single company. By April 2002, as already noted, negotiations were already in progress (with 'the first sur-

*This policy is to change in future, as described in the Postscript.

gical teams having been brought in from abroad').[11] A national planning exercise involving the 'local health economies', announced by the DH, began in May of that year.

Wave 1 ISTC contracts were initially planned and negotiated by the Department of Health's National Implementation Team (NIT), which seems to have existed from at least as early as 2002. In June 2003, however, the Department created a Commercial Directorate with a specific remit 'to introduce Independent Sector Providers to the NHS'.[12] The Commercial Directorate was defined as 'the central point in securing best value as well as achieving greater levels of effectiveness for the Department and the National Health Service through the use of best commercial practices and better commercial relationships. It is also responsible for the procurement of independent sector treatment centres and the implementation of the NHS supply chain excellence programme'.*[13]

The first Commercial Director, Ken Anderson, was an American who had joined the Department of Health in November 2002 from Amey, a company involved in PFI projects, where he was Director of Health Services, and would leave it again in 2006 to become Managing Director and Vice Chairman of the Swiss bank UBS. In 2004 Anderson told an interviewer:

We act as an interface with the independent sector and ensure that organisations can engage in a commercially ap-

---

*The National Implementation Team and the Commercial Directorate also employed a large number of outside management consultants: In the financial year 2004–05, the directorate used the following consultancy and legal firms at a cost of £38.4 million, including £12.8 million on legal advice, from the department's programmes' budget. These were: Accenture Plc., Addelshaw Goddard, Ashurst and Co., Atos Origin IT, Augmentis, Avail/Yale/Tribal Consulting, Currie and Brown, Deloitte, AT Kearney, Eversheds, Freshfields Bruckhaus Deringer, Gardiner and Theobald, HOK International, KPMG, Marsh UK Ltd., Morgan Cole, National Economic Research, NDY Consulting, NHS Professionals, OVE Arup and Partners, Precept, PriceWaterhouse Coopers, Translucency Ltd., Willis Ltd., Wragge and Co (Commons Hansard Written Answers 18 Jan 2006: Column 1409W). At least two of these had a prima facie conflict of interest; Tribal Consulting belonged to the Tribal Group which owned Mercury Health. Mercury Health eventually won six of the first wave contracts, comprising ten ISTCs. Atos Origin IT was part of a group which was later awarded the second largest diagnostic contract in Phase 2 of the programme. The contract was cancelled in 2007 for substandard performance.

propriate way. My team and I hail from the private sector so we understand commercial and procurement issues. We are not afraid to look closely at deals and arrangements with private sector suppliers and partners to ensure we get the very best value. However, it is not all about driving down prices, because we are also making it easier for independent organisations to deal with the DH and NHS. That may be in speeding up the procurement process, simplifying procedures or encouraging organisations to innovate and try new ideas.[14]

b) The procurement process

The procurement process was to be 'efficient, effective, and fast', and would typically be in three stages – 'a short-listing process; submission of detailed bids, resulting as soon as practically possible (and after determination of a price) in the identification of a preferred bidder; finalizing of project details (where both sides have committed to take the project forward)'.[15] But Wave 1 was also supposed to be based on local assessments of the need for extra capacity. In written evidence to the House of Commons Health Committee the Department of Health described the process as follows:

In October 2002, the Department conducted an extensive forward planning exercise, during which all Strategic Health Authorities (SHAs) were asked to identify, in conjunction with their respective Primary Care Trusts, any anticipated gaps in their capacity needed to meet the 2005 waiting time targets. The result of this exercise led to the identification of capacity gaps across the country, particularly in specialities such as cataract removal and orthopaedic procedures, where additional capacity was needed beyond the increased capacity planned by existing NHS providers. As a consequence, a procurement exercise was launched. In December 2002, the Department invited expressions of interest from the independent sector to run a series of Treatment Centres, in order to enable yet more NHS patients to benefit from faster access to surgery.[16]

Or as Mr Anderson told the Committee: 'The process that we went through was one where we would go out to the local NHS through the strategic health authorities and ask them what capacity gaps they had and what they could not accomplish or provide themselves either efficiently or at all. The primary objective was the capacity issue'.[17] This statement was strongly disputed. It is discussed further in Chapter 2, in relation to both capacity and choice.

(c) The terms of ISTC contracts

The DH's 'ISTC Manual',[18] updated in December 2006, states that 'all the contracts are based on a single generic model contract' to facilitate the 'agreement of standard commercial terms with the IS whilst minimizing the need for costly and lengthy negotiations'. It is not known when this generic contract was introduced. The key provisions of Phase 1 ISTC contracts were foreshadowed in the 'Growing Capacity' documents of June and December 2002; others emerged in subsequent information presented in Outline Business Cases (OBCs) and 'redacted' Full Business Cases (FBCs) obtained by the authors. The provisions were:

(i) **Contracts run typically for five years** from the date of commencement of services (i.e. excluding any construction period that may be involved).

(ii) **Contracts are for a specified number of completed procedures**, defined as 'finished consultant episodes' (FCEs).

(iii) **Guaranteed volumes of work.** Phase 1 contracts are based on guaranteed volumes of clinical activity for the ISTC provider, known as the 'Minimum Take' (also often referred to as 'Take or Pay'). The provider is paid for the contracted number of procedures, whether or not all of them are carried out. According to the ISTC Manual this was necessary 'in order to benefit from the competitive pricing structures that the providers are thus able to offer';[19] i.e. ISTC providers could offer lower prices per procedure if they did not carry the risk that the specified number of patients might not be forthcoming. Payments are fixed annual amounts, paid in monthly instalments, and 'each individual Sponsor (PCT or NHS Trust) is responsible for a proportion of the Minimum Take' – i.e. the commissioning PCTs or Trusts which are parties to the contract must between them ensure that a minimum number of patients are referred to the ISTC; if not they must pay for them anyway.* If a Sponsor is unable to make any payment due under the terms of the contract, the Secretary of State will make the payment on its behalf.[20] In other words, 'demand risk' is entirely borne by the NHS.

(iv) **Clinical standards.** All professional clinical staff 'must appear on the appropriate register of their professional body', and 'all doctors must appear on the specialist register for their specialty'.[21] ISTC providers must ensure that clinical governance arrangements are in place. Responsibility for performance management is assigned to a Joint Service Review and a Contract Management Board, both of which are ultimately reviewed by the Commercial Directorate.[22]** Providers are obliged to submit data on Key Performance Indicators (KPIs) on a monthly basis, the information to be validated on a quarterly basis by the National Centre for Health Outcomes Data (NCHOD). This information is to be used 'to benchmark Provider performance against like-for-like care providers'.[23] If, following investigation by the Joint Service Review, there is a 'threshold breach' of a KPI by an ISTC provider, 'a rectification plan may be drawn up, outlining expected

*PCTs which are not parties to the contract can also make referrals to the ISTC via one of the PCTs which is a party, if this is necessary to ensure that the number of referrals meets the monthly 'Minimum Take'. Contracting PCTs may also buy 5% more procedures than the total in the contract, which the Provider must supply. Additional clinical activity above this figure can also be undertaken following negotiations between the parties.

**The JSR consists of the Provider, the Sponsor(s) and the Contract Manager. The CMB consists of the Sponsors and Contract Manager and reports to the Head of the Central Contract Management Unit arm of the Commercial Directorate. JSR and CMB issues ultimately come to the Programme Board of the Central Clinical Procurement Programme in the Commercial Directorate.

actions by the Provider within a stated time frame'. If this plan is not implemented 'the Contracts allow for the Sponsors to impose financial penalties', and in 'extreme' circumstances the ultimate sanction is contract termination.[24]*

(vii) **Clinical performance risk.** The ISTC Manual states that 'The general position is that the Provider is responsible for dealing with any problems and the costs arising from them. If the Provider does not have the facilities or staff to deal with a specific problem, the Provider must arrange a transfer to a healthcare provider with the appropriate facilities, usually the local NHS Acute Trust. This position is reflected in the Associated Costs payments which the Provider must pay in the event that a procedure goes wrong or a patient reacts badly to surgery'.[25] The amounts involved in such payments are not known. The risk of lawsuits for clinical negligence, however, is in principle assumed by the NHS. Since July 2004 ISTC providers have been able to benefit from the Sponsor's membership of the NHS Litigation Authority's (NHSLA) Clinical Negligence Scheme for Trusts (CNST), which means that if patients make claims for medical negligence, the CNST will cover the costs of any such claims.

(viii) '**Additionality**'. The rule that ISTCs must supply additional resources was a key element of contracts in Wave 1, which was primarily justified in terms of 'increasing the current clinical and human resource capacity of the NHS' by 'using human resource capacity which is genuinely in addition to that available to Health Service Bodies...' Recruitment from the NHS would act as a drain on its staffing capacity 'and defeat the purpose of the ISTC programme as a whole'.[26] Phase 1 ISTCs were therefore barred from employing any healthcare professional employed by the NHS in the previous 6 months.

---

*If a serious incident occurs a Joint Service Review must be convened to identify the cause of the problem. Following recommendations on how to deal with the incident, 'the Provider is assisted in developing an action plan'. Providers are also required to report incidents to the Healthcare Commission under section 28 of the Care Standards Act 2000, as amended by the Health and Social Care Act 2003.

Certain exemptions were allowed, however. The most significant was local secondment of NHS staff to ISTCs. According to the DH, 'IS Treatment Centres also handle some activity that has been transferred at the request of the local NHS to free up capacity in existing facilities for other important clinical activity. In these cases, existing NHS staff can operate in the units on a structured secondment basis to ensure there is no dilution of existing NHS staff and resources'.[27] While this policy of 'structured secondment' is ostensibly adjusted according to local requests, its implementation was soon co-ordinated at a national level. The NHS Employers' 'Human Resources Framework for Wave 1 ISTCs', published in January 2005, said that a 'national framework has been developed to support the secondment of staff to ISTCs'. On average 25 per cent of the clinical staff of the 23 Wave 1 ISTCs have been drawn from the NHS.[28] In some ISTCs the proportion is much higher: in Waltham Forest ISTC, for example, 83 per cent of the staff are seconded from the NHS.[29]

General Supplementary contracts

The private provision of elective procedures by Wave 1 ISTCs has been supplemented by some additional procedures purchased from 'incumbent' private providers (i.e. the established British private hospital operators, chiefly BUPA and Nuffield) through a series of 'General Supplementary' (known as 'G-Supp') contracts, and some smaller regional block contracts – 'short-term contracts to meet the government's long-term 18 week maximum waiting time target by 2008'.[30] In 2003 the DH announced plans to contract at least 125,000 extra operations over 5 years in this way – i.e. an average of at least an additional 25,000 procedures a year. For 2004/05 28,400 orthopaedic procedures, costing £74.5million,[31] were contracted for with Capio Healthcare and Nuffield Hospitals, and in May 2005 a £54 million contract for 13,500 orthopaedic procedures was made with three independent providers: the General Healthcare Group (5,000 procedures); Nuffield (5,000 procedures), and BUPA (3,500 procedures). The market analysts Laing and Buisson thought, however, that 'this second G-Supp [might] well be the last as the government does not see a long-term need to continue this type of contracting, with ISTCs the preferred procurement model... although the DH has not completely ruled out further use'.[32]*

Independent Sector Treatment Centres: Phase 2

In March 2005 the Department of Health began a second phase of national procurement of independent provision. In 2006 it told the Commons Health Committee:

> Phase 2 Electives is expected to deliver up to 250,000 procedures per year and create an Extended Choice Network (ECN) of Independent Sector Providers who will deliver up to an additional 150,000 procedures per year, on an *ad hoc* basis. Overall, this represents an investment of approximately £3 billion over five years... Phase 2 Diagnostics is expected to deliver approximately two million additional diagnostic procedures per year for NHS patients, and represents an investment of over £1 billion over five years.[33]

The total annual proposed Phase 2 electives figure of 400,000 may be compared with the 5.6 million elective procedures which the DH estimated were being carried out by the NHS in 2006.[34] The companies and areas involved for Phase 2 ISTC contracts at the beginning of 2007 are shown in Table 3. (The status of Phase 2 in mid-November 2007 is described in the Postscript).

*Laing and Buisson also noted that 'In addition to G-Supp some independent hospital groups have won a handful of smaller regional contracts'.

Table 3
Phase 2 Electives contracts (services commencing in 2007 or 2008) under negotiation in January 2007

SCHEME	COMPANY	TYPES OF PROCEDURE	NO. OF ROCEDURES# P.A.
Tyne and Wear	BUPA	General	5,000
Cheshire and Merseyside	BUPA	General	16,800
Cumbria and Lancashire	Netcare	CATS*	160,000
Avon, Gloucestershire and Wiltshire	UK Specialist Hospitals	General	27,800
Cumbria and Lancashire	Capio	General surgery	15,000
London North	Clinicenta	CATC*	221,000
London South	Clinicenta	CASS*	299,000
West Midlands	Nuffield	General	29,324
Essex	Mercury Health	General, rehab	29,000
Greater Manchester (A)	Netcare	CATS*	44,000
Greater Manchester (B)	Care UK	CATS*	44,000
Hampshire/Isle of Wight	Partnership Health Group	General	123,300
England	Fresenius	Haemodialysis	100,000
Total			**1,114,224**

The numbers of procedures are approximate. They are also indicative only, as they comprise assessments, diagnoses and diagnostic tests as well as surgery, rehabilitation treatment, etc.
*CATS – Clinical Assessment, Treatment and Services; CATC – Community Assessment Treatment Centre; CASS – Community Assessment Support Spoke.
Source: Department of Health, 'Phase 2 Electives and Diagnostics Update', January 2007.

The DH's statement to the Health Committee laid little stress on the Extended Care Network of private providers, and the Committee's Report made no mention of it. A year later it would

emerge that more NHS patients were expected to be treated by
the ECN than by ISTCs. In Chapter 3 we will see just how important this is.

Changes in the nature of ISTC contracts for Phase 2

At the time of writing (September 2007) very little information
was available about Phase 2 contracts. In comparison with Wave
1, however, three main changes are being made.

First, the additionality rule has been relaxed to allow Phase 2
ISTCs to employ any NHS staff who are not in 'shortage professions'; and they may also employ NHS staff in shortage professions in their 'non-contracted hours' – 'if you like, their overtime
hours', the General Counsel to the Commercial Directorate told
the Health Committee.[35] The Department of Health summed up
the new policy as follows: 'Additionality will not apply to NHS
employees except those included in the list of shortage professions and will apply for all NHS employees in respect of their non
contracted hours'.[36] The list of shortage professions was amended
substantially in August 2007, following a review undertaken by a
body attached to Hampshire and Isle of Wight SHA, responsible
for analysing NHS workforce data.*

Second, Phase 2 contracts still include 'Minimum Take' ('Take
or Pay') clauses, but these are intended to be 'tapered'. The clear-
est statement of what this means was given by the then Secretary
of State, Patricia Hewitt, to the Health Committee:

> As we move to a system of patient choice it will be the pa-
> tient who decides where they actually go. The real issue
> here, I think, is risk. Do we ask new providers or independ-

*The specialties and professions removed from the additionality list were: Clinical radiol-
ogy (consultants); Biomedical scientists; Therapeutic and diagnostic radiography - bands
6 and below; Trauma and orthopaedic surgery (consultants); Occupational therapists;
Otolaryngology (consultants); General surgery (consultants); Gynaecology (consultants);
Ophthalmology (consultants); Physiotherapy; Urology (consultants); Gastroenterology
(consultants); Medical physics and engineering (HCS); Anaesthetics (consultants); Plas-
tic surgery (consultants); Respiratory medicine (consultants); Rheumatology (consultants); Neurosurgery (consultants). [Email communication from Andrea Hester, Head of
Programmes, NHS Employers, 10 September 2007]

ent sector providers to invest in facilities and simply do that on the basis that if they get the patients they get paid, and if they do not get the patients, they do not? Now, that will mean transferring the entire risk to those providers and that is likely to cost more than if we share some of that risk. Obviously with the take or pay contracts, really we carry the whole of the risk and that is why you can look at variations between all of the risk being held by the Department, all of the risk being held by the contractor or the risk actually being shared, so we have asked providers to bid on the basis of tapering guarantees for contracts because we think that will be much more appropriate in Wave 2...What we want to get to is by the end of the initial guaranteed contract period all independent sector providers should be providing service obviously of NHS quality, but also at the equivalent of NHS tariff...*37

A third change is that Phase 2 contracts include a routine option to build in training. Bidders were asked to bid for contracts with and without the provision of training. The effect of taking on training would be to reduce substantially the number of cases that could be dealt with in a day. No figures for the extra cost of this have been provided.

The combined effect of these changes, and the greater 'integration' between ISTCs and local NHS providers called for by the Health Committee and most of the clinicians who gave evidence

* The DH written submission to the Health Committee stated that 'Phase two contracts will be based only on indicative volumes of procedures in recognition of the introduction of patient choice. Providers have been asked to bid on the basis of tapering guarantees for contracts... the intention being that IS providers should all be providing services at NHS tariff equivalent by the end of the initial guaranteed contract period in line with the level playing field and free choice'. [House of Commons Health Committee Report on Independent Sector Treatment Centres, Session 2005-06, Vol II, Ev. 10] According to *Healthcare Market News*, October 2005, in Phase 2 contracts 'the DH will guarantee a proportion of activity which will gradually diminish over the term of the contract. Interestingly, the DH seems to be using this as a negotiating mechanism saying that it will present the "maximum" level of activity it is willing to guarantee, which will be the same for each scheme, in the invitations to negotiate and invite providers to propose lower levels as part of the negotiation process'.

to it (discussed in Chapter 3), was to point to a situation in which for-profit providers would be operating in a market alongside NHS providers, and on increasingly similar terms. Whether for-profit providers could make profits if the 'playing field' was truly levelled, and what the impact would eventually be on NHS trusts and foundation trusts affected by the competition, remained to be seen.

Conclusion

By June 2007 ISTCs were in existence across the whole of England, plus one in Scotland. They had been allowed to call themselves 'NHS Treatment Centres' and use the NHS logo, so that from the point of view of patients they were indistinguishable from treatment centres operated by NHS trusts, and appeared to be part of the NHS. The distinction between Wave 1 for-profit providers, dealing with low-risk cases at much higher cost than NHS providers, and NHS trusts, was no longer clear. The level of performance actually achieved by Wave 1 ISTCs is discussed in Chapter 2.

Notes

1 Department of Health, *The NHS Plan: a plan for investment, a plan for reform*, Cm 4818-I, July 2000.
2 Department of Health, *Delivering the NHS Plan: next steps on investment, next steps on reform.* (Cm 5503 April 2002, p. 28).
3 Freedom of Information response from the Department of Health, DE00000189579, 27 March 2007.
4 Department of Health, *The NHS Plan: a plan for investment, a plan for reform*, Cm 4818-I, July 2000.
5 Cm 5503, April 2002, p. 27 (6.2).
6 Department of Health, *Growing capacity: a new role for external healthcare providers in England* (June 2002, p.3).
7 Ibid., p.6.
8 Department of Health. *Growing capacity independent sector diagnosis and treatment centres*, December 2002.
9 Ibid., p 10.
10 HC Report, Vol II, Ev. 1.
11 *Delivering the NHS`Plan: Next steps on investment, next steps on*

reform, Cm 5503, April 2002, p. 27 (6.2).

12   Department of Health, '*Working with the Commercial Directorate – A Guide to Commercial Commissioning*' (2006, p. 4).

13   Commons Hansard: 18 Jan 2006: Column 1408W.

14   Association of British Healthcare Industries, 'Innovation through procurement: driving innovation in the NHS through the procurement process: An interview with Ken Anderson', *Focus Magazine* (2004).   www.abhi.org.uk/multimedia/downloads/2006/ARwebsite1.pdf

15   Department of Health, *Growing capacity independent sector diagnosis and treatment centres*, December 2002, p. 7.

16   HC Report, Vol II, Ev. 1.

17   HC Report, Vol III, Ev. 1.

18   Department of Health, *ISTC Manual Independent Sector Treatment Centre (ISTC) Programme*, February 2006. Alternative title: ISTC Wave 1 Manual Gateway reference: 6136.

19   ISTC Manual, p. 25.

20   ISTC Manual, p. 31.

21   ISTC Manual, p. 52.

22   ISTC Manual, p. 51.

23   Ibid.

24   Ibid.

25   ISTC Manual, p. 32.

26   ISTC Manual, p. 23.

27   Department of Health, 'Treatment Centres: Delivering Faster, Quality Care and Choice for NHS Patients', January 2005, p. 10.

28   Freedom of Information response from the Department of Health, DE00000180956, 21 February 2007.

29   Waltham Forest NHS Primary Care Trust, *Independent Sector Treatment Centre (ISTC) – Update*, 22 May 2005.

30   Laing & Buisson. Laing's Healthcare Market Review, 19th Edition 2006/2007, p. 17.

31   Laing & Buisson, 'Capio lands £9.6m NHS deal', *Healthcare Market News*, November 2004.

32   Ibid,, p.113.

33   HC Report, Vol II, Ev. 1.

34   HC Report, Vol II, Ev.. 2.

35   HC Report, Vol III, Ev. 107.

36   The Government's Response to the Health Committee's Report on Independent Sector Treatment Centres, Cm 6930, October 2006, p. 13.

37   HC Report ,Vol III, Ev. 98.

CHAPTER 2: ASSESSING THE ISTC PROGRAMME – THE HEALTH SELECT COMMITTEE'S ENQUIRY

The first systematic attempt to review and assess the ISTC programme was made by the House of Commons Health Committee from March to July 2006, and offered the first extended opportunity for Parliament to hold the Department of Health (DH) to account for the policy. In this Part we review the Committee's enquiry and its results, which can fairly be described as somewhat inconsistent and inconclusive. Above all the Committee failed to address the fundamental aim of the ISTC programme, i.e. to help create a healthcare market, focusing instead on a series of more specific claims made for it by the DH. One witness, Professor John Appleby, chief economist at the Kings Fund, came close to spelling out this central aim, suggesting that the high cost of ISTCs was really the price paid for bringing a market into being:

> From a Department of Health point of view, one of the aims, the vision, it seems to me, is market creation: it is to fit in with the more pluralistic provider supply side and a desire, frankly, to put pressure on, and, in a sense, destabilise the NHS – not completely, of course, but to ginger up the market, if you like, with the independent sector. I guess that to entice them into this potential market, compromises were made on both sides, in terms of finances and the nature of the contract that was on the table...[1]

But the Committee either did not grasp the importance of this observation, or declined to pursue it. The terms of reference it set for itself did not assign priority to the issue of competition, and the evidence given to it by the DH referred to it only obliquely, as will be seen below. Moreover the answers given to the Committee by the Department's Commercial Director, Ken Anderson, and its Head of Demand Side Reform, Bob Ricketts, who were primarily responsible for the programme, were often – and as some Committee members noted, at times deliberately – uninformative. The DH also refused to supply the Committee with any financial information, or with any precise details of the formula which had been used to evaluate the value for money (VFM) of ISTC providers' bids, on the grounds that to do so would disclose commercially confidential information and would jeopardise the government's future bargaining position with private providers.[2] In its report, however, the Committee conformed to tradition by responding to these and other obstacles that limited its investigation only with relatively mild expressions of concern.

The Committee began by trying to identify the goals of the programme against which it should be assessed:

> The ISTC programme has had a number of objectives, but it has proved surprisingly difficult to identify them or establish the weight given to each of them since a different emphasis has been placed on different objectives at different times. The Government's broad goals seem to have been to use the ISTC programme to: increase capacity; reduce spot purchase prices in the private sector; increase choice; introduce best practice and innovation and diffuse these through the NHS; and through the challenge of competition from ISTCs, stimulate reform and improve efficiency in the NHS (the "grit in the oyster" argument).[3]

But, the Committee added,

> In our final evidence session with Department of Health Officials we were told of another objective for the ISTC scheme: to assist reconfiguration; for example, existing hospitals might be closed and some of the facilities replaced by an ISTC.[4]

But this clue to the longer-run aim of the ISTC programme was presented as applying only to Phase 2, and was not in practice followed up by the Committee.

We examine the Committee's treatment of each of the first set of objectives in turn, although (for ease of exposition) not in quite the same order. We also combine the objectives of 'introducing and diffusing best practice' with 'the challenge of competition'; and that of lowering spot prices with the closely-linked question of value for money, which was also one of the HC's terms of reference, and on which they actually spent more time. We look at the data and comment on the Committee's treatment of it in each case.

Increased capacity

a) *Wave 1*

How far has the ISTC programme increased the NHS's capacity to deliver care?

It is important to note from the outset that there are strictly speaking no data of any kind on ISTC capacity, in terms of either staff or beds, nor did the Health Committee ask for any. Given the aim of bringing in additional 'medical professionals' and increasing capacity it is curious that in response to a request for data, the Information Centre for Health and Social Care said, 'At present we do not collect workforce data from ISTCs although we are discussing with the Department of Health how this might happen for the next census in September 2007'.[5] Workforce data were also unobtainable from the Commercial Directorate. Similarly, in response to a request for data on bed numbers in treatment centres, the DH replied, 'Nothing is required from Independent Sector Treatment Centres'.[6] In terms of bed availability, the Commercial Directorate said, 'bed availability in the ISTCs is not collected as ISTC beds do not form part of the bed capacity available to the NHS'.[7]

Instead, 'capacity' has been consistently understood as being represented by the numbers of procedures contracted for and performed. The DH told the Committee that Wave 1 ISTCs were 'expected to provide an average of over 170,000 Finished Consultant Episodes (FCEs) a year over five years' (a total of 850,000) for 'an investment of approximately £1.6 billion'.[8] This statement did not distinguish between elective and diagnostic procedures; but while the DH told the Committee that Wave 1 ISTCs had performed 'over 9,000 diagnostic procedures for NHS patients', in fact a total of 912,000 diagnostic procedures over five years was contracted for.[9]

No routine data are published on ISTC performance, either; what exists are aggregated figures for all types of procedure and all ISTCs which have been disclosed in response to a parliamentary question or an FOI request, or provided to the Health Committee or the Healthcare Commission. Table 4 provides all the information available down to July 2007.

Table 4

Procedures said to have been carried out by Wave 1 ISTCs down to April 2007: cumulative totals

	1	2	3	4	5
	To Dec 2005*	To Apr 2006**	To Jan 2007***	To April 2007#	To April 2007##
Electives	44,000	59,960	107,000	128,000	167,850
Diagnostics	9,000	25,151	60,000	73,000	307,435
Total	53,000	85,111	167,000	201,000	474,870
Primary Care			11,679		140,485

Sources
* Department of Health, evidence to the Health Committee, *Independent Sector Treatment Centres*, Fourth Report of Session 2005-06,,Vol II Ev. 1.
** Answer to Parliamentary Question by Andrew Lansley MP, Commons Daily Hansard, Written Answers, 13 July 2006: Column 2062W.
***Department of Health Response to Freedom of Information request, DE00000189579, 27 March 2007.
Data supplied by the Department of Health in response to FOI request, DE00000241293, 22 October 2007.
##Data supplied by the DH to the Healthcare Commission and published in its report, *Independent Sector Treatment Centres: Review of the quality of Care*, July 2007, p. 6.

But these figures are problematic, and reveal a significant degree of divergence between the number of procedures reported by the DH to the Healthcare Commission and those obtained through an FOI request a few months later.

First, according to the Healthcare Commission's figures shown in column 5, the total number of electives performed up to April 2007 was 167,850, compared with the total of 128,000 obtained via a Freedom of Information (FOI) request. The discrepancy is due to the fact that 'the ISTC programme figures supplied to the Healthcare Commission include elective procedures... done under the G Sup 1 and 2 contracts...'. [10] In other words, the Healthcare Commission's figure is inflated by some 40,000 procedures (167,850 minus 128,000) which were carried out by non-ISTC private providers, but are now counted as part of 'the ISTC programme'.

Second, the even more substantial increase in the number of diagnostics apparently carried out between January and April 2007 – 247,000 (column 5 minus column 3), after a previous total of 60,000 in three years – turns out also to be due to the fact that the figures supplied by the DH to the Healthcare Commission included diagnostic procedures carried out by providers under G-Supp and 'pathfinder programmes'. By the end of April 2007 ISTCs had actually only carried out 'more than 73,000' diagnostic procedures.[11] The Healthcare Commission's figure thus inflates the actual ISTC performance of diagnostic procedures by 234,000, or 420 per cent.

Third, in its written presentation to the Health Committee the DH had made no reference to ISTCs being contracted to provide primary care. The procedures which it said it expected to be provided were 'Finished Consultant Episodes', not procedures performed by 'GPs, community and practice nurses, community therapists' (the official definition of primary care). In its written submission the DH mentioned that one centre, in Portsmouth, included a 'walk-in centre/minor injuries unit', but the words 'primary care' were used nowhere in the memorandum. In response to the above-mentioned FOI request, however, the Department stated that 'within the ISTC programme primary care is delivered through six commuter focused walk-in centres and one ISTC, which has a minor injuries unit and walk-in centre'.[12] The consultations taking place in these centres are 'procedures' included under 'primary care' in the bottom row of Table 4. No explanation was offered for treating these walk-in centres as 'within the ISTC programme'.

The data given to the Healthcare Commission by the DH and shown in column 5 of Table 4 thus seriously overstate the performance of ISTCs, and the Commission's statement that 'by 30th April 2007, 615,771 patients had undergone procedures at ISTCs'[13] is untrue.

The Health Committee had itself been sceptical of the DH's figures. It thought that even the figure of 60,000 FCEs which the DH told them were being carried out by ISTCs in 2006 might have been inflated by the inclusion of non-ISTC activity.[14] It also noted that 'the Department pointed out that 250,000 patients had been treated or diagnosed in the independent sector by the end of 2005'. But, the Committee said, 'only a minority of these – 50,000 – were treated in the mainstream ISTC programme, the rest representing independent provision of procedures not in the ISTC programme such as MRI scans'.[15]

Attempts to inflate the figures ultimately only serve to underscore the fact that performance has fallen drastically short of the expected average of 170,000 elective procedures a year. In relation to the 5.6 million elective procedures estimated to be carried out by the NHS in 2006,[16] the true ISTC figure was minimal. The Committee concluded that 'ISTCs have not made a major direct contribution to increasing capacity', noting that the Department had admitted as much.[17]

Indeed the Health Committee was concerned to know whether, as numerous NHS witnesses claimed, the ISTC programme, however modest, also represented an unnecessary addition to capacity, and whether it was destabilising some NHS trusts and treatment centres. It noted that the West Hertfordshire Hospitals NHS trust would lose about £15 million as a result of the establishment of an ISTC in Hemel Hempstead.[18] Each of the six PCTs in the Northumberland, Tyne and Wear Strategic Health Authority had to contribute £200,000 a year for five years to pay for the contract negotiated with Capio UK to run an ISTC in their area; three of them had fewer than 100 patients treated by the ISTC, and one of them only fourteen.[19] In another example, at a time when a financial crisis was imposing cuts in other services, South West Oxfordshire PCT had had to pay Netcare £255,000 in the first six months of its contract to provide cataract operations, even though, thanks to the 'Take or Pay' clause in its contract, it performed work to a value of only £40,000 during the period in question.[20]

But while individual examples of unnecessary 'additional' capacity were noted, the Committee was not told about, and did not investigate, the extent of 'transferred activity' – activity transferred from NHS trusts – within the total numbers of procedures carried out by ISTCs. According to NHS Employers, the workforce arm of the NHS Confederation (the organisation of NHS managers), such activity resulted from

> a short-term overlap or redistribution of the existing clinical activities in the acute trusts and the planned activities in the treatment centres. In the medium to long-term, this "transferred activity" will enable the acute trust to refocus resources in other areas of need. In the short-term however, detailed work on staffing by some acute trust hospitals involved in the programme will involve use of NHS staff on a secondment basis.[21]

As already noted, some 25% of the staff working in ISTCs in Wave 1 were on such secondment arrangements, and there is a correlation between the figures for seconded *staff* and those for transferred *activity*. A DH document states that

> Providers will be able to use NHS staff when providing the Services for Schemes where there is transferred activ-

ity. Where there is transferred activity it is expected that the amount of NHS staff time available to the Provider (as a proportion of the Provider's total staffing requirement) will be approximately equal to the amount of transferred activity as a proportion of total activity to be delivered by the Provider.[22]

In other words, as of February 2007 approximately 25% of all work carried out in Wave 1 ISTCs was not additional work but 'transferred activity'; work that would have been carried out by NHS trusts but was instead given to ISTCs and performed there by NHS staff. Meanwhile, so far from being short of capacity, some NHS Treatment Centres had actually been closed for lack of demand. A well-known example is Ravenscourt Park in west London. It was bought from BUPA in 2002, but by August 2006 it had to close, having attracted 'only half the patients it needed for viability'.[23] Projected losses of £37m were forecast by 2010, 'because of high running costs and lack of demand'.[24] The solution adopted was to sell the centre back to BUPA. But to make this possible, patient demand had to be raised. The North West London Strategic Health Authority ordered several NHS trusts, including North West London Hospitals NHS Trust and Chelsea and Westminster Healthcare NHS Trust, to transfer 1,500 cases per year to Ravenscourt Park, doubling its throughput.[25] Part of the restructuring plans included the use of the proceeds of the sale of Ravenscourt Park to form a joint venture with BUPA to build and run a new private oncology centre at Charing Cross Hospital. The management was transferred to BUPA, although the NHS had to continue paying for the remainder of the lease.

A second example is the Central Middlesex Hospital's Ambulatory Care and Diagnostic Centre (ACAD), the first NHS 'fast-track' diagnosis and surgery centre, which opened in 1999. Initially hailed by Tony Blair as the 'embodiment of the new NHS', by November 2004 the centre was running at 50% capacity and faced closure after losing more than £3.4m in potential revenue. The Deputy Chief Executive of Central Middlesex Hospitals,

Mark Devlin, expressed frustration that the Trust had 'not been able to use the ACAD facilities fully because taxpayers' cash is flowing to the private sector. The London Patient Choice caseload is most at risk from the independent sector diagnostic and treatment centres'.[26]

Some trusts have refused to reveal whether NHS Treatment Centres for which they are responsible are operating with spare capacity or at a loss.* In response to an enquiry, Newham University Hospital NHS Trust, London, for example, would say only that 'The capacity of the Gateway Surgical Centre is constantly under review'.[27] Many NHS Treatment Centres are, however, experiencing problems relating to capacity. These include Dartford & Gravesham(Kent); Brunel (Swindon); Cannock Chase (Mid-Staffordshire); Ravenscourt Park (London); Huntington (Cambridgeshire) and Good Hope in the West Midlands. Hinchingbrooke, for example, is 'deeply in debt, partly because of the centre's failure to generate predicted levels of income'.[28] Far from attracting extra patients from wider catchment areas, many NHS TCs, such as Dartford and Gravesham, are not attracting sufficient numbers of local patients. Others, such as Cannock Chase, have seen their income diverted to neighbouring ISTCs. Cannock Chase NHS Treatment Centre was opened in 2003 to tackle ophthalmology and orthopaedic waiting lists. 'Then', according to *Hospital Doctor*, 'an ISTC was opened 25 miles away at Queen's Hospital, Burton. A Mid Staffordshire Trust spokesman says the NHS centre is now operating with 60 per cent spare capacity in orthopaedics and 40 per cent in ophthalmology. "Work which was originally going to Cannock then went to Burton", he says'.[29]

The Committee concluded that

*Some NHS TCs listed by the Health Committee are apparently not called Treatment Centres by the NHS Trusts responsible for them. For example King's College Hospital is not only listed in the report, but also appears on the DH website as a 'pioneering practice example' of an NHS treatment centre. The website refers to the hospital's 'new treatment centre facility' carrying out its first prostate treatment in April 2003. However a trust spokeswoman claims to know nothing about it. 'We have a day surgery unit, but that was opened in 1992', she says. The Royal Cornwall Hospitals NHS Trust, which also appears on the list, similarly admits to having a day surgery unit, but was unaware that it had been characterized as 'Truro treatment centre'. (*Hospital Doctor* 5 November 2006).

ISTCs have not made a major direct contribution to increasing capacity, as the Department of Health has admitted. It is far from obvious that the capacity provided by the ISTCs was needed in all the areas where Phase I ISTCs have been built, despite claims by the Department that capacity needs were assessed locally.[30]

Two comments are necessary at this point. First, the Committee did not comment on the general significance of the fact that the total of £1.6 billion committed to Wave 1 (and the further £4 billion committed to Phase 2, discussed below) comes out of existing NHS funds – the budgets of the PCTs making the contracts, and the DH's central budget (PCTs pay the equivalent of the NHS tariff for the contracted procedures, the extra cost of the contract price being covered by the DH under what is known as the 'Dual Tariff'). Any capacity created in ISTCs was thus never a net addition to the NHS's overall capacity. In other words the Health Committee did not consider the opportunity cost of the £5.6 billion diverted to ISTCs. Given the difference between the NHS tariff and the cost of procedures contracted from ISTCs (let alone the cost of those actually performed, which under the 'Take or Pay' provision in their contracts could be far below the number contracted for), there was a net loss of capacity, not a gain.

Second, the Committee heard extensive evidence showing that the 'local NHS' had not been significantly involved in capacity planning, and thought this might well have led to capacity being created in some places where it was not really needed. It did not comment on the significance of the fact that this was systematic: negotiations with providers were initiated long before even the local outposts of the NHS Executive, let alone local NHS clinicians, were consulted.

Mr Simon Kelly, speaking for the Royal College of Ophthalmologists, rejected the DH's claim that capacity planning had been decided locally. Mr Ian Leslie, the president of the British Orthopaedic Association, told the committee that 'there was no collaboration with the professionals who knew something about

hip replacements and how they are done during the early times…
The involvement of the orthopaedic world was very scant'.[31]
The NHS Alliance, representing all those involved in delivering
primary care, told the Committee that 'The lack of widespread
clinical engagement with local GPs and NHS hospital consultants
has been a significant failure of the first wave of ISTC procurement'.[32]

A non-executive board member of South-West Oxfordshire
PCT, Jane Hanna, told the Committee:

> in Oxfordshire the non-executives were very concerned
> that any views of local professionals which were expressing
> concerns about the treatment centre, whether it was needed
> and issues of quality and impact on local services, were kept
> away from the [executive] board. That did not just include
> local specialists who were providing the NHS service, it in-
> cluded the optometrists in the local community who wrote
> to the chief executive asking for information to be placed
> before the board expressing their concerns that by transfer-
> ring activity from the eye hospital to the private provider it
> would seriously prejudice training and would impact nega-
> tively on quality of clinical services for the future. They were
> expressing concern that they were very happy with the local
> service and it was looking to meet target and, therefore, why
> was the change being made to an unknown provider. That
> piece of paper was simply not shown to the board. The local
> impact statement by the specialist at the eye hospital was
> not shown to the board before we made our decision, even
> though the non-executives were constantly asking for infor-
> mation about local impact.[33]

A glance at the chronology of the capacity planning process shown in the Box below makes it clear why there was in fact
no significant local involvement in capacity planning. The time
given to the Strategic Health Authorities, not to mention PCTs,
to produce capacity plans of a kind that had never been undertaken before was manifestly too short, and at that early stage in

BOX: CAPACITY PLANNING FOR THE ISTC PROGRAMME IN 2002 – CHRONOLOGY

28 March 2002: Margaret Edwards, Director of Access & Choice at the Department of Health, writes to Strategic Health Authorities (SHAs) asking them to prepare and send 'Capacity Plans' to DHSCs (Directors of Health and Social Care) by mid-June.

2 May 2002: An SHA Chief Executives Board Meeting says 'further clarification of what was expected in capacity plans would be helpful'.

10 May 2002 The same request is made by DHSC Directors at an Access Board meeting.

14 May 2002: Bob Ricketts, DH Head of Capacity and Choice, writes to DHSC Directors asking them to 'identify a substantial number of sites within your DHSC area for using overseas clinical teams to supplement capacity *substantially* [emphasis in original] and to make significant, and sustained, inroads into long waiting times'. 'First mover sites' are to be identified by 29 May, and Ministers 'have signalled that they want to see a substantial number of schemes developed in 2002/03 with as many of these as can be safely delivered coming on stream by the end of July this year, with others coming on stream in the following months'.

16 May 2002: In response to the SHA Board Meeting of 2 May Margaret Edwards sends guidance entitled 'Capacity Plans: Clarifying Expectations', which 'has been prepared for use by DHSCs with SHAs'. Edwards acknowledges that 'the development of whole system capacity plans represents a major challenge for SHA and PCTs at an early stage in their development and when many have not yet got a full complement of staff... Nevertheless to deliver the NHS Plan access targets we need to begin to build up the momentum for capacity expansion and service redesign now. Furthermore we will be agreeing with you key investment decisions (e.g. for the sites for the second wave of DTCs, new day surgery facilities, use of European teams) in mid-July, informed by the initial capacity plans'. A document by Bob Ricketts accompanying the 'Capacity Plans' guidance states that 'This is the first time that a systematic capacity planning process has been carried out by the whole NHS, linked to delivering clear medium-term targets', and there 'is an urgent need to accelerate planning and delivery of the extra capacity needed to meet the key access targets'. Capacity plans are to 'be summarised for each year to show the respective contributions to additional activity from additional NHS elective capacity, overseas/independent sector, DTCs, use of beds freed up from day cases, increased day case rates, additional NHS emergency capacity, contribution from reducing delayed transfers of care and reducing emergency admissions'.

The expected timetable for the planning process is given in the guidance as follows:

30 May 2002: Agreement reached on the timetable and process for assessing capacity plans. 'SHAs which envisage serious difficulties in meeting the March 2003 targets must have informed their DHSCs so that discussions can take place during June about options'.

30 June 2002: 'Capacity Plans submitted by SHAs to DHSCs, copied by DHSCs to Bob Ricketts in the Access Directorate'. By this date confirmation was also expected on a common methodology for modelling demand and supply to be agreed and disseminated for developing capacity plans for 2003/04 to 2005/06.

31 October 2002: 'SHAs submit definitive capacity plans for 2003/04 – 2005/06 to DHSCs, copied to the Access Directorate'.
Source
Department of Health Response to Freedom of Information request, DE00000241505, 25 October 2007.

the evolution of SHAs and PCTs the skilled resources to do such planning often did not exist. As for serious participation by local clinicians, it was clearly out of the question. It is clear that the National Implementation Team, and subsequently the Commercial Directorate, worked out an overall programme in negotiations with prospective providers and then secured local agreement, where necessary by the exercise of considerable pressure.

b) *Phase 2*
In spite of the Committee's conclusion that Wave 1 had not contributed to capacity, and its scepticism that it had been needed in the areas where ISTCs were established, it accepted the DH's assurances that the need for an additional 400,000 elective procedures and 2,000,000 diagnostic procedures (later reduced to 1,500,000), to be performed annually by ISTCs and other private providers in Phase 2, had been assessed locally. By June 2006, the Department said, it had expected these procedures to be provided by 22 new ISTCs, but the number was reduced by seven because they were not all needed. The Committee saw this reduction as 'suggesting a degree of local influence' in capacity planning. It did later comment that 'The decision to maintain the commitment

to spend £550 million per year [on Phase 2] despite changing circumstances [i.e. the seven withdrawn schemes] has not been explained, and seems to sit uncomfortably with the Secretary of State's admission that "in other [areas] it has become clear that the level of capacity required by the local NHS does not justify new ISTC schemes".[34]

But while seven of the ISTC schemes originally proposed had been withdrawn, the DH was also negotiating with bidders for seven 'regional diagnostic schemes' covering the whole of England. The Committee listed these in its report, but made no further reference to them. At least some or these would later emerge as CATS or ICATS, which were clearly about 'assisting with reconfiguration' – the late addition to the DH's list of functions for the ISTC programme, mentioned earlier, and discussed in Part 3 below.

The Health Committee was concerned that lack of integration between ISTCs and the NHS was inefficient and therefore welcomed the relaxation of the additionality rule for Phase 2, recommending that the DH 'should ensure that Phase 2 contracts encourage NHS staff to be seconded to treatment centres'. The Committee further recommended that NHS consultants should be allowed to hold sessions of planned activities in ISTCs 'where this would be thought appropriate for local service needs and to aid integration'.[35]

But it did not remark on the staffing implications of the numbers of procedures being contracted for under Phase 2. If it had proved hard to get enough non-NHS staff for Wave 1 ISTCs to provide a total of just 128,000 elective procedures and 73,000 diagnostic procedures (the total numbers actually carried out by April 30 2007 – see Table 3, above) over more than 3 years – let alone the average of 170,000 elective procedures and 182,400 diagnostic procedures *per year* contracted for – where were staff to come from to provide the 400,000 additional elective procedures a year, and 1.5 million diagnostics, contemplated under Phase 2? The Committee did not mention any numbers in its report, but a moment's thought makes it obvious that these additional procedures could not be provided without relying on NHS staff, on a scale that could hardly be managed on the basis of 'ad hoc' or even 'structural secondments'. In effect, the plans for Phase 2 implied the extensive transfer of NHS staff to private sector employment. The significance of this is taken up in Chapter 3.

Innovation and best practice

To the Health Committee the DH maintained that ISTCs embody best practice and innovative techniques, and were driving these throughout the NHS. To the market, however, it admitted that it 'had been disappointed by the level of innovation present in Wave 1 contracts and was looking for real innovation and different service models for the second wave'.[36] Innovations identified by the DH included the use of mobile units to improve access; blood conservancy and recycling methods; and wider use of local rather than general anaesthesia.[37] But witnesses from the Royal Colleges of Ophthalmology and Orthopaedics, and from the BMA, stressed that these practices were already followed in the NHS. The Committee observed that 'Innovation in ISTCs is largely a matter of better processes and clinical management rather than surgical techniques or technological advances. It is probable that it has been driven by the regular case-mix and stems from the "elective surgery only" character of all treatment centres rather than by the independent sector's involvement in the treatment centre programme'.[38] Of course, since a quarter of ISTC clinical staff were seconded from the NHS, it was hardly surprising that the surgical techniques and technology used tended to be the same.

It is significant that the DH's claims to the Committee about the objectives achieved by such innovative methods did not include higher productivity. An earlier claim to that effect had been shown to be an extreme case of spin. In January 2005 the DH claimed that 'In the IS Treatment Centre programme, each of the mobile cataract units is performing an average of 39 cataract removals per day during their visits to selected parts of the NHS... In 2002-03 the NHS in England carried out more than 270,000 cataract removals in 141 different providers. This equates to about five cataract removals per provider per day, which contrasts with the 39 removals per day in the mobile cataract units'.[39] In a departmental press release a month later this became, 'Research has shown that independent treatment centres are performing operations at eight times the rate of the NHS due to modern, purpose-built units concentrating on single procedures'.[40]

The spin was successful. For example the CBI's director of public services declared in May 2005 that, 'Critically, it [the ISTC programme] introduces a powerful set of incentives to raise productivity across the sector as a whole. Early evidence suggests that the use of treatment centres has stimulated a five to eight times increase in the productivity of cataract operations'.[41] The President of the Royal College of Ophthalmologists responded: 'Surgeons in independent treatment centres are not a super race, able to perform cataract surgery at up to eight times the rate of their NHS counterparts… It is NHS eye surgeons who have dramatically cut waiting times with small incision day-case cataract surgery. They also perform a whole range of other complex procedures and teach and train as well'.[42] But in July the Conservatives' shadow Chancellor could still say that 'independently run NHS treatment centres… now treat up to eight times as many cataract operations a day than (sic) the NHS has traditionally managed'.[43]

Inside the DH, however, a warning light seems to have come on.* In a report to the Secretary of State in February 2006 Ken Anderson reduced the productivity claim by almost half: 'The report highlights productivity and efficiency gains that independent sector treatment centres have pioneered, such as: mobile

*In order to ascertain the nature and validity of the productivity claim we asked the DH for a copy of the research mentioned. After several weeks, following reassurances that efforts were being made to find it, a formal FOI request was sent. The response gave a spreadsheet for the NHS figures for the year 2002-03 but offered no figures for the ISTCs. Instead it stated, 'The figure of five cataract removals per day was derived from Hospital Episode Statistics (HES). It is difficult to make a like-for-like comparison between providers because most of the cataract operations done within NHS organisations are in units which perform other procedures during each day, whereas, as the press release states, the mobile cataract treatment centres focus on carrying out high volumes of a single procedure'.

units capable of delivering up to 20-23 ophthalmology cases per day due to streamlined procedures enabling efficient use of theatre space and surgical resource'.[44]

But in the meantime serious issues of quality had emerged concerning these mobile ophthalmology units, owned and operated by Netcare. Some of them had been staffed by foreign surgeons on very short visits to the UK, and by their nature mobile units could not provide any significant follow-up. Netcare's medical director, Dr Dinesh Verma, was appointed in April 2004 but resigned in October the same year. According to *Hospital Doctor*, he 'repeatedly raised concerns about on-call cover, continuity of care and access to complete outcome data for audit'.[45]

So the Committee was concerned to know whether the quality of the work done at ISTCs was as good as that done in the NHS, rather than whether it was better. But this it found impossible to establish. The Key Performance Indicators, or KPIs, which ISTCs are contractually obliged to collect, largely concern process issues such as cancellations, the average duration of induction, procedure and recovery, and patient satisfaction rates. Observing that only 8 of the 26 KPIs were clinical indicators of any kind, the Committee said the Department should have ensured that comparable clinical data were collected from both NHS and private providers, and published, in order accurately to assess quality of care, complication rates and other quality measures.

Daniel Eayres, giving evidence for the National Centre for Health Outcomes Development (NCHOD), which had undertaken the first research on the quality of the ISTC programme,[46] went much further; he said that only one KPI, number 15, could be considered as a 'pure clinical outcome indicator'. KPI 15 includes 'complication rates and wound infections, but also patient–reported outcome measures, where the status of the patient is measured before the operation and the status of the patient is measured again after the operation and some sort of measure of improvement or change or impact is made'. But for KPI 15, he added, 'no data has so far been collected and given to us':[47] in every data set received from the first group of ISTCs reviewed by

NCHOD, KPI 15 was marked 'not applicable'.[48]

Other problematic data issues identified by NCHOD included late delivery of data; substantial additional work because of the poor quality of the data; mismatched data arriving from different sources within the DH; substantial variation in the interpretation of the definitions of some KPIs; and variation in data collection and completeness. There was also the fact that NCHOD was unable to validate the data: Eayres told the Committee: 'We are basically accepting what the ISTC give us. They say, "Oh yes, we had 100 admissions, five of those led to readmissions". They give us that; we cannot really validate it at the moment'.[49] These difficulties taken as a whole rendered 'any attempt at commenting on trends and comparisons between schemes and with any external benchmarks futile'.[50] The Health Minister, Lord Warner, by contrast, saw the KPI data as 'heartening" evidence of "a robust and comprehensive quality assurance and reporting system'.[51]

The Chief Medical Officer had in the meantime requested a review of the quality of care in ISTCs from the Healthcare Commission. The terms of reference were modified, in light of the Health Committee's criticisms, to make clinical quality its key focus, and its report was published in July 2007. The Commission put the best gloss possible on the evidence, saying that 'This review provides some positive assurance about the quality of care provided by ISTCs', pointing to evidence that 'care pathways are designed to meet the needs of patients, and patients rate their care highly', and that 'processes of care appear to function well'.[52]

> We have analysed the national data sets, and although the data are provisional and there remain problems with the quality of data collected by ISTCs, indicators such as the rates of emergency readmission to hospital and length of stay in hospital suggests that ISTCs have lower rates than NHS establishments for most procedures reviewed.

It noted, however, that

This is in keeping with their mix of patients, which excludes those with the most complex health needs.... But data on diagnosis and procedure... need to be collected routinely to make any assessment and these data are currently of poor quality.[53]

And it went on to confirm the judgment of the NCHOD in all respects. As most commentators at the time noted, the Commission's key finding was that it could not properly assess the quality of care in ISTCs because the necessary information was lacking:

There have been longstanding problems with the completeness and quality of HES [Hospital Episode Statistics] data from ISTCs... it is only very recently that the completeness of data submitted is starting to reflect their volumes of activity. The quality of the data submitted was also, until recently, too poor for meaningful analysis.[54] There were no identifiable data from some ISTCs for some periods; only seven ISTCs could be identified in the 2005-2006 data, and only nine in the data for the first six months of 2006-2007...By the third quarter of 2006-2007, the position had improved and only two ISTCs were not submitting data. Where HES data were submitted by ISTCs, while the quality of data was good in a number of fields, it was poor in some important ones....[55] We are concerned about the lack of high quality, routinely-available, systematically collected data on individual patients that is essential for the assessment of the processes and outcomes of care.[56]

Moreover 'The Department of Health did not until very recently enforce the contractual requirement for ISTCs to submit high-quality data to the HES, nor did it make such submissions a priority'.[57] In future, the Commission said, the data collected from ISTCs and other independent providers of services to NHS patients should be 'the same as that submitted by the NHS, allowing comparisons to be made'.[58] The Commission reported that it had received evidence from professional bodies about clinical outcomes in ISTCs, but did not indicate that it had investigated this evidence.

In lieu of valid evidence on outcomes the Commission laid considerable stress on the results of a patient satisfaction survey it had conducted, which showed that ISTC orthopaedic patients were significantly more satisfied with the treatment they had received than equivalent NHS patients. The Commission acknowledged, however, that it had not been able to control entirely for the possible effects of differences in case mix and 'other factors'. It did not comment on the possible effects of the most obvious 'other factor', namely that the price paid per patient actually treated in ISTCs was so much higher than for those treated by the NHS. That would presumably be relevant to many of the differences, such as the fact that 100 per cent of ISTC patients reported that enough nurses were on duty, compared with only 90 per cent of NHS patients, etc.

Given the lack of valid official data on the clinical performance of ISTCs, it is reasonable to ask what other information is available.

The Health Committee noted that 'A significant number of witnesses, including patients and professional bodies, criticized the quality of care provided to patients by ISTCs'. Problems cited included the use of foreign-trained surgeons, who were unfamiliar with NHS processes and surgical techniques, and language difficulties. As late as November 2003, when the first ISTC was already operating, concerns were expressed over the staffing of ISTCs, with some doctors warning that there would not be enough suitably qualified surgeons and anaesthetists to carry out the number of procedures promised by the DH. An article in *Healthcare Market News* reported that:

Although the ISTC plan has already reached preferred bidder stage, the precise rules covering the grade of doctor operating in both NHS and ISTCs remain unclear. James Johnson, chairman of the BMA Council, told HMN that

as far as he is aware, the rules covering doctors working in
ISTCs have yet to be finalized. Indeed high-ranking DH
officials themselves do not know what the rules will be, he
said. Johnson said he was shocked when one DH official
told him that while surgeons working in ISTCs will have to
be on the specialist register, anaesthetists will not. A spokes-
person for the NCSC [National Care Standards Commis-
sion] said that, at the very least, overseas doctors working
in ISTCs will have to be on the specialist register, something
Johnson said would be an "insuperable problem". "Getting
all these doctors, especially from overseas, on the specialist
register, would be extremely difficult".[59]

Additionally, the Health Committee noted,

Some surgeons working in ISTCs, albeit a decreasing
number, have come to the UK to work for a weekend or
a few weeks, and are therefore often unable to follow up,
or even be aware of, complications... ISTC providers stated
that the level of complications and unexpected transfers
back to NHS facilities were low... Many others disagree. In
evidence to the Committee, the BOA [British Orthopaedic
Association] claimed that orthopaedic surgeons working
in the NHS had seen above-average revision and re-admis-
sion rates for patients who had been treated in ISTCs. They
claimed that there were revision rates of 2.3% in ISTCs, compared to only 0.7% in the NHS. The organisation described
stories of "overseas surgeons inserting unfamiliar prostheses, not cementing those designed to be cemented etc". The
Royal Colleges and the BMA also voiced concern about the
quality of care in ISTCs. The Royal College of Surgeons of
England told the Committee of "increasing evidence" that
ISTCs were unable to manage complications "with conse-
quent transfer to existing NHS facilities and on occasions to
the consultant to whom the patient was initially referred".[60]

In December 2005 the BMA undertook a survey of 91 clinical directors in the three specialties – anaesthetics, ophthalmology and orthopaedics – chiefly involved in Wave 1 ISTCs, to assess the ISTCs' impact on the 'local health economies' in which they were located.[61] In terms of clinical quality the report found that '(a) Half of respondents express concern about the general quality of care provided by treatment centres overall, but with significantly greater concern regarding the quality of care in ISTCs than in NHS Treatment Centres: (b) Over 80 per cent of respondents say that there was either no formal arrangement for reporting concerns regarding patient care and clinical governance to ISTCs, or that they are unaware of it'. Many clinicians also reported a 'high turnover of consultants working in the treatment centres' with its impact on continuity of care; others mentioned the lack of information provided to them 'as to the qualifications of surgeons employed' who appear to be accredited on a 'fast-tracking' basis.[62]

Mr Ian Leslie, the president of the BOA, agreed that the available clinical evidence was 'anecdotal' but thought there was

> now enough evidence gathering out there. My colleagues see the bad results coming back. Bad results perhaps in eye surgery and hernia surgery occur rapidly. In orthopaedic surgery, they occur over five years, maybe 10 years, so we are seeing dislocation rates and revision rates, and if one is seeing that with our patients, it is no wonder we are being negative about the way it is being done.[63]

The BOA, he said, had submitted two dossiers of cases to the Department of Health.

> The first went to then deputy chief medical officer Aidan Halligan about 16 months ago and the second was submitted nine months ago... Although they investigated, it hasn't made much difference to our concerns... The difficulty is getting hold of the information from the ISTCs. But in two centres where the figures have been examined the failure

rate was significantly higher than in NHS hospitals - at a diagnostic and treatment centre in Weston-super-Mare it was
three times the NHS rate and in Cheltenham it was something like 10 times the rate.[64]

The Professor of Orthopaedic Surgery at Nottingham University, Professor Angus Wallace, wrote in the *BMJ* that the 'number
of patients we are seeing with problems resulting from poor surgery [in ISTCs] is too great'; with the NHS 'being left to pick up
the pieces'. The problems identified were 'incorrectly inserted
prostheses, technical errors, and infected joint replacements'. In
addition,

> The single supplier contracts that most ISTCs use also
> means that only one joint replacement type is available to
> the surgeon and that is the one that he or she is asked to put
> in. It's clear that this has occurred with inadequate training
> of both the surgeons and the operating theatre staff and as
> a consequence there have been several serious errors – e.g.
> joint replacements put in without bone cement when bone
> cement was essential for that joint replacement, the use of
> incorrect size heads (ball) for a hip joint replacement.[65]

In an interview with the *Guardian* Professor Wallace added:
'We expect failures of hip replacements at approximately 1% a
year and knees at about 1.5% a year. But we have got some of the
ISTCs that are looking at 20% failure rates'.*[66]

---

*In a 'Rapid Response' exchange in the *BMJ* a management consultant asked if he were
'the only person reading this who is concerned by the lack of statistics to back up the
claims made'? adding, 'This is an important debate and should not be primarily decided by anecdotes from a not exactly disinterested source'. In response Professor Wallace
said the respondent was 'quite right. It is important to have comparable statistics. The
British Orthopaedic Association approached Aidan Halligan, the Deputy Chief Medical
Officer at the Department of Health, about 15 months ago and asked for an independent comparative audit of outcomes from joint replacement operations to be carried out.
This was so the Treatment Centres and NHS Hospital outcomes could be compared in
order to monitor the quality of treatment in both. This was initially agreed; the audit
was planned but was subsequently suspended. We do not know why'. (*BMJ*, Rapid Response, 'Comparable Statistics Required', 17-19 March 2005. http://www.bmj.com/cgi/
eletters/332/7541/614#130038)

Another orthopaedic surgeon, Gordon Bannister, 'compared 1,754 joint replacement operations at the [NHS] Avon Orthopaedic Centre with 137 performed in the Cheltenham Nuffield [ISTC]. The Nuffield's re-operation rate for knee replacements was ten per cent, compared with the NHS' one per cent. For hips it was 12 per cent, compared with 0.7 per cent in the NHS'.[67]

Eye, the Journal of the Royal College of Ophthalmologists, published two early reports on ISTC projects that offered some data. The first found that the incidence of presumed infectious endophthalmitis (PIE) in Bolton Hospitals NHS Trust was both clinically and statistically different from that in the Lancaster Netcare (ISTC) unit. Three cases of PIE out of 929 eyes undergoing cataract extraction were found in Lancaster (Netcare) compared with 7 out of 12,831 in Bolton.[68] The second report, published in 2005, noted that 'the audit of cataract surgery outcomes from Lancaster in 2002 is still awaited despite the outbreak of endophthalmitis occurring in that early Netcare initiative'.[69]

Netcare's orthopaedic ISTC in Portsmouth was the subject of a review commissioned by the Hampshire and Isle of Wight Strategic Health Authority, following allegations about the same company's operations at MoD Royal Hospital Haslar. Following a BBC report on 29th April 2004, Portsmouth Hospitals NHS Trust confirmed that concerns had been raised about the quality of five hip replacement operations carried out by one surgeon at Haslar. The Trust said that all operations undertaken by this surgeon, as well as hip replacements performed by other Netcare surgeons, would be reviewed to ensure they were of a 'standard equitable to the NHS'. The review found that timescales were 'ambitious given the numbers involved and the mix of cases'. Concerns over clinical standards were raised during the contract after post-operative complications. There were poor procedures to recruit doctors, who were described by Netcare as their 'associates', rather than their employees; Netcare considered itself to be an 'introduction agency' and believed it to be Portsmouth Hospitals NHS Trust's responsibility to satisfy itself that the Netcare surgeons were competent. Vetting procedures for Netcare's surgical team were described as 'weak', and references were 'not always seen'. While Netcare's audit procedures were described as 'of a high quality', they measured surgical outcomes only until the patient was discharged, not over the longer term.*[170]

To conclude on the issue of quality: the fact that after more than three years there were still no data on clinical outcomes that could be compared with those of NHS hospitals and treatment centres was treated by the Health Committee as a merely unfortunate difficulty. It said that the DH should have collected such data from the outset, but did not insist on it being collected forthwith, and it omitted to criticise the DH for not insisting that data for KPI 15, the sole KPI that directly concerns clinical outcomes, were reported.[71] On the other hand the Committee expressed strong criticism of the British Orthopaedic Association's 'questionable claim' that there are revision rates of 2.3% in ISTCs, and dismissed as unreliable most of the evidence it had received of shortcomings in the clinical standards of some ISTCs.**[72]

*The law firm Michelmores has several clients who have brought cases of malpractice against Netcare at MoD Royal Hospital Haslar in Portsmouth. Michelmores argue that the SHA report, which had to be obtained through an FOI request, 'fails to probe far enough into the issues surrounding Netcare's provision of outsourced surgical procedures', with a 'concern that private providers, under pressure to drive down costs, may be tempted to cut too many corners'. The report, while drawing attention to the issues mentioned above, more or less 'exonerates the company'. But as Michelmores point out the reference frame for the report was only a 10-day period, which in the context of a 6-month period [the period during which Netcare had undertaken procedures at Haslar] 'cannot represent a thorough analysis of the events that led to our clients' injuries'. The narrow remit also focuses on the activities of a single doctor, ignoring the performance of the other Netcare surgeons. The cost of the procedures was another cause for concern, and Michelmores ask, 'Whether Netcare was under pressure to deliver a range of orthopaedic procedures with varying complexity and risk factors too cheaply'. The SHA report also fails to mention that the Netcare surgeons were not registered on the GMC's specialist register ('Haslar Report "a missed opportunity" claim Michelmores'. http://medneg. michelmores.com/netcare/orthopaedic-page1.asp)

**The question of quality has not been restricted to ISTCs. A report by the BOA on the lack of quality assurance in operations outsourced to the private sector includes work done by Nuffield and Capio under G-Supp contracts. The BOA president, Michael Benson, who subsequently requested a DH investigation, said 6 overseas surgeons working on fast-track initiatives had been suspended for surgical errors. 'We asked that all overseas surgeons be evaluated and assessed by the college or Specialist Advisory Committee, as NHS consultants are. That request has been ignored'. The report also found systems failures, with patients referred to the private sector being rejected as too complex or unfit. Mr Benson said one was transferred between five surgeons before being placed back on the NHS waiting list. He added: 'We have no idea how many complaints there have been, what the audit structure is, or what patient outcomes are'. ('Quality under attack', *Hospital Doctor* 19 May 2005.)

On this issue the Health Committee appeared effectively to col-
lude with the DH. ISTCs are treating NHS patients, for whom the
NHS has a duty of care, with procedures involving serious risks,
and the 'Minimum Take' element in their contracts gives PCTs a
very strong incentive to try to ensure that the requisite number of
patients are treated by the ISTCs they have contracts with. Given
this, the failure of the DH to ensure from the outset the collection
from ISTCs of exactly the same clinical outcome data as are collected by the NHS seems plainly culpable.

Increased choice

The extension of choice in healthcare became a central theme of
government policy in health care from 2001 onwards, and the
DH claimed that extending choice had been a central aim of the
ISTC programme from the outset. Its written submission to the
HC stated:

> The ISTC programme will play an important role in imple-
> menting patient choice. Patient choice is being introduced
> in stages... Currently around a third of PCTs' choice op-
> tions include the independent sector (ISTCs and other IS
> providers). Choice at referral will benefit some 9.4 million
> patients by meeting their needs and preferences.   During
> 2006, choice will extend to include NHS Foundation Trusts,
> all centrally procured ISTCs and other subsequently cen-
> trally procured independent sector providers. By 2008, pa-
> tients will be able to choose to be treated by any healthcare
> provider that meets NHS standards and can provide care
> within the price the NHS is prepared to pay.[73]

A King's Fund paper published in 2005 noted that choice has
many facets: it is seen as a way of 'meeting patient expectations,
improving efficiency, reducing waiting lists and strengthening local accountability'.[74] In relation to ISTCs, however, choice was
compromised at more than one level. This was especially the case
in respect of the choice of alternative providers of treatment that

is offered to patients, and the choice offered by the DH to local health care planners, in so far as they represented the local community.

As regards the first, the Health Committee noted that where the establishment of an ISTC led to the closure of NHS facilities, patients would have no more choice than before. It also noted that in the absence of clinical outcome data, patients – and GPs – could not make an informed choice of elective care providers.[75] But it failed to comment on the fact that the 'Take or Pay' ISTC contracts created a powerful financial incentive for PCTs to ensure that patients chose to use ISTCs rather than NHS providers, since the PCT had to pay the ISTC whether it performed the contracted number of procedures or not. If patients chose not to use the ISTC, the PCT had to pay the NHS provider which supplied the treatment as well. A few PCTs even offered GPs a financial payment for every patient they referred successfully to an ISTC for elective treatment, a measure of the financial loss to the PCT if the 'slots' at the ISTC were not taken up. For example in 2006 Tameside and Glossop PCT offered GPs £130 for every patient referred to Netcare's Greater Manchester Surgical Centre – a significant raise over the £30 per patient previously offered by Ashton, Wigan and Leigh PCT to send patients to the same place, and a measure of how much the failure of GPs to refer patients for treatments which the PCT was already obliged to pay for was costing the PCTs with which Netcare had the 'Take or Pay' contracts.[76]

The second way in which the ISTC programme reduced choice rather than extending it has already been touched on: the contradiction between the central procurement of ISTCs, and official commitment to local participation in decision-making about whether an ISTC was needed – or wanted. At the Labour Party Conference in September 2003 then Health Secretary John Reid had said, 'We will decentralize the control and power over local commissioning, through PCTs and over local hospitals through foundation status. We'll give local people the chance to control their health providers'. But by the time most boards of PCTs and local clinicians were informed of the DH's intention to establish a local ISTC, negotiations were well advanced. PCT managers were seen as privy to the plans, but non-executive board members and local NHS staff usually seem to have been informed only when contracts were close to being signed. In written evidence to the Health Committee Dr Sally Ruane, an academic, noted that a *Health Service Journal* survey of over 100 NHS chief executives found that 'the programme was being forced through by "bullying", making a mockery of local choice':

> The imposition of centrally negotiated schemes in locations, determined perhaps by the preferences of the commercial operator regardless of local performance and capacity, with potential damage to the local health economy has attracted vehement criticism from PCTs, Trust chief executives, NHS`Elect and the NHS Confederation. The events surrounding the alleged imposition of a Netcare scheme specialising in cataract work in Oxfordshire and its impact on the viability of the local highly regarded NHS eye unit, compounded by the subsequent failure of Netcare to perform contracted procedures, have attracted widespread critical press coverage and been the cause of scandal.[77]

The clear impression given by the evidence of the chief witness in this particular case, Jane Hanna, a lawyer and former non-executive board member of the South West Oxfordshire PCT, is that the PCT managers saw their careers as being in jeopardy if they failed to get the non-executive members of the board to endorse a decision already taken by the DH. In this instance, because the Oxford Eye Hospital was highly rated and on track to meet the government's waiting time target, the non-executive members of the PCT could see that there was no local need for an ISTC, and that its 'Take or Pay' contract would mean that the Eye Hospital would be financially destabilised. They therefore voted not to sign the contract.

Ms. Hanna told the Committee:

> The ... evidence indicated there was no need for a treat-
> ment centre in our area and, therefore, we were concerned
> that given that the strategic health authority was looking to
> bring the decision forward at that time that we would be
> looking to vote "no" at the board meetings because the evi-
> dence would not be in place. At that point we were threat-
> ened with a personal surcharge by managers at the strategic
> health authority.[78]

After the decision was made not to proceed with the ISTC contract,

> all the non-executive directors were called by the chair of
> the PCT and were told that he had been told that John Reid
> [the Secretary of State for Health] wanted a reversal of the
> decision on his desk by 12 o'clock on the Monday. The
> words that were used to us were that Jane Betts of the SHA
> was on the way to the NHS Appointments Commission and
> the tables were turning, by which we all understood that our
> positions as non-executive directors were under threat. The
> chair had previously told us that he had been informed that
> two other chairs of boards had been told that they would
> lose their jobs if their boards voted against the treatment
> centres.[79]

Ms Hanna also referred the Committee to a statement by Jane
Betts, the chief executive of the local Strategic Health Authority. Ms Betts said: '...it became clear to me that on the issue of
the treatment centres my role and that of the board and the executives had been completely subsumed to the will of Richmond
House [the DH offices in Whitehall]. This placed my staff in great
distress and made my board impotent. We became a conduit for
communication rather than being able to handle the issue ourselves'.[80]

Not all PCTs resisted the imposition of ISTCs, and no other PCT seems to have gone so far as to refuse to sign the required contract. But the evidence is very clear that the plans were made with little local consultation, and where necessary imposed. Choice in the matter of whether there should be a local ISTC was not on offer.

Value for money

'Value for money' or VFM was not one of the objectives of the ISTC programme listed by the DH for the Health Committee, although it had been one of the main aims cited in the Department's June 2002 prospectus, *Growing Capacity: A new role for external providers in England*, which said ISTCs were to attain 'High value for money: the productivity levels of such units will be such that they can offer services at competitive unit costs',[81] and the claim was regularly repeated in official documents, statements and press releases throughout Wave 1.[82] But the Health Committee's terms of reference included VFM, and after assessing the government's related claim that ISTCs had the objective of reducing the 'spot prices' charged by the 'incumbent' private providers (Nuffield, BUPA, and others), the Committee spent a good deal of time on VFM.

On spot prices – the prices paid by NHS trusts for purchases of procedures from private providers as and when they were needed, which the DH said had been 'upwards of 40% over reference costs' (now the NHS tariff)[83] – oral evidence given to the Committee claimed that they had fallen. One witness, the chief executive of Mendip PCT, said they had fallen in his area by as much as 50%.[84] This was an interesting claim, since unless they had previously been at least twice as high as tariff; a 50% fall meant that they must have fallen to less than tariff. Had that been the case, the chief executive would presumably have remarked on it, since the claim that ISTCs will eventually compete at the NHS tariff is a key part of the government's case. Ken Anderson, for example, told the Health Committee that 'if private providers cannot compete at tariff once that is instituted then they will not be providing the care to patients'.[85] So either Mendip had previously been paying exceptionally high prices to private providers or the DH's statement that spot prices had been 'upwards of 40%' above tariff was an understatement.

Since on the most favourable assumptions ISTCs had by then contributed about one percent of total elective and diagnostic capacity, a general fall in spot prices was not due to the contribution of ISTCs. The Secretary of State told the Committee that there was now 'no real need to use spot purchasing at all',[86] due presumably to the expansion of NHS capacity and the fact that purchases from private hospitals through the 'G-Supp' contracts were now being made in bulk (with corresponding unit cost reductions).[87]

The question of value for money (VFM) was more sensitive. The Committee wanted to know whether an adequate assessment of VFM was made before the bids were accepted, and whether the Wave 1 ISTC programme had provided VFM. The Committee was unable to get answers to either question, because the DH refused to provide any financial information about the contracts signed, or any precise detail about the methodology it used in assessing VFM; or about the results of an independent review it had commissioned to ascertain whether the methodology used was being consistently and correctly applied (the DH said the review had found that the methodology was being used consistently and correctly, but still refused to show the review to the Committee).[88] The Health Committee was also apparently refused evidence on VFM in a closed session with Ken Anderson and Bleddyn Rees, General Counsel to the Commercial Directorate, following the final hearing.[89] In a later BBC Radio 4 interview, the Health Committee's Chairman, Kevin Barron, was asked about the problems associated with obtaining information from the DH:

> **Interviewer:** Let's look now at the question of value for money. You say you can't assess this because the Department of Health won't give you the detailed analysis of the figures that's needed.

Barron: Yes, absolutely right. I would have liked to have seen them, but in real terms we did not get the detail and actually what we did in the report, we said the National Audit Office ought to look at it. They do have a department that will and can go in there and understand the issues around money.[90]

In general Barron showed a marked disinclination to complain about the Government's lack of evidence but was eventually provoked in the same interview to say, '...quite frankly, if evidence is there then why the hell didn't they give it to us?'

In the absence of the information denied to the Committee we can only make a series of observations on what the DH said about VFM.

The DH accepted that the fact that ISTC prices were less than the former spot prices hardly represented VFM by comparison with NHS provision, but it maintained that the premium above NHS Equivalent Cost did represent VFM. In a supplementary memorandum to the Health Committee the DH outlined its VFM methodology in general terms as follows:

An NHS Equivalent Cost is calculated for each scheme and compared against the bid price. The percentage variance between the two is known as the VFM of the scheme.

Independent sector providers face costs which are not borne by the NHS such as staff recruitment to comply with the additionality rules, establishment costs (for example the funding of new builds), the costs associated with bidding, and of direct taxation (including corporation and value added tax). These additional costs that are borne by providers are the reason why a premium above the NHS Equivalent Cost has been necessary.

A VFM threshold above the NHS Equivalent Cost was set at a level substantially lower than the prevailing spot rates – with no schemes progressing that showed VFM above that level. The average achieved for Wave 1 is 11.2% in comparison with the historical "spot-purchasing" rates of in excess of 40% above NHS Tariff.*

The NHS Equivalent Cost is a calculation of the amount that would be paid to an NHS provider for delivering the same activity in the same location as the provider with the same care pathway. It is necessary to provide a baseline against which bids from the independent sector can be compared.

NHS Equivalent Cost is derived from NHS National Tariff (which is based on average costs within the NHS for providing clinical procedures) with specified adjustments to reflect the IS provider's delivery model (including restrictions on the type of patient that can be admitted), the cost of outpatient appointments etc, anticipated inflation rates and the Market Forces Factor ("MFF") that would apply for NHS providers in that (geographic) health economy.[91]

This statement poses several puzzles. First, given that at the start of the ISTC programme 16 NHS Treatment Centres were already in existence, the question arises why VFM could not be calculated by comparing ISTC costs with theirs. The Health Committee actually pressed the Health Secretary on this. The answer was noticeably evasive:

Chairman: Why was it not possible to use NHS Treatment Centre programmes as a comparator?
Ms Hewitt: There were very few of those at the time we embarked upon this, I think I am right in saying.
Chairman: But there were some.
Ms Hewitt: We are talking about a period before my time and I am afraid I have not got all that detail with me.
Chairman: I realise that. It is possibly not directly a ques-

---

*This statement is ambiguous – does it mean 11.2% above tariff or 11.2% above NHS Equivalent Cost? Most readers have assumed the latter (e.g. *Public Finance*, 28 April 2006), but the alternative reading seems equally valid.

tion to you, Secretary of State, but there were some. We would just like to know why it was not the case that they were used.

Sir Ian Carruthers [Acting Chief Executive of the NHS]: In essence, NHS Treatment Centres were very often part of individual hospitals and their costing structures actually were very similar to the NHS main hospital provision. So I think that very often they were additions to the facilities that ran in an ordinary way. I think we can look at that but the reality is that that will be consumed in most of the costs of normal hospital provision because I think treatment centres were quite often in many instances just extensions of the local hospital.

Chairman: Are you looking at them differently now? We were actually in one last week. It may be on the same site as a hospital and adjoined to the building but it is run differently from the hospital.

Ms Hewitt: I think, if I may say so, that reflects part of the change that is happening within the NHS. One of the problems that arose in the old, if you like, more monolithic NHS, is that actually there was not great transparency about costs and the NHS did not, in the old days, have a very good understanding of the costs of doing different kinds of procedures in different kinds of places....[92]

The Committee let that go.

They also failed to question the meaning of the 'NHS Equivalent Cost'. NHS Equivalent Cost would appear to play something of the same role that the Public Sector Comparator or PSC plays in VFM calculations for PFI projects, where the cost of a notionally equivalent public sector project is calculated, and then the cost of the risks supposed to be borne by the private sector provider are added to it; the private option is adopted when it appears better value for money. The PSC is notional, both in not being based on the costs of an actually existing public sector institution, and in being costed on the basis of various costs that the private provider is assumed to face, which differ from those of an NHS provider. This leaves a lot of room for manoeuvre, in which the private provider can be made to appear to offer better VFM.* NHS Equivalent Cost would appear to play a similar role in calculating VFM for ISTCs.

Nor did the Committee question the rationale for paying a premium above the NHS Equivalent Cost, based on the need to cover extra costs borne by the private sector provider of an ISTC. Paying for the costs of bidding, for example, only makes sense if there are more than equivalent benefits to be obtained from procuring services through a bidding process (the market-creation aim alluded to by Professor Appleby in his evidence to the Committee cited earlier), but the Committee did not pursue this. The inclusion in the premium of the cost of 'new builds' is also curious. Not only do NHS trusts also have to pay for their new builds, but the DH also undertakes to buy any new buildings put up by an ISTC at the end of its contract if the contract is not renewed.[93] In that situation it appears at first sight as if the NHS will have paid for them twice.

Some individual Full Business Cases which have been obtained show that risk transfer featured significantly in them. The full business case for the East Lincolnshire ISTC, for example, includes the following 'risk allocation matrix':

*How the PSC may be manipulated to produce the conclusion that a PFI procurement is better value for money than public procurement was demonstrated clearly in the case of the Haringey secondary schools. See Melanie McFadyean and David Rowland, 'PFI vs Democracy? School Governors and the Haringey Schools PFI Scheme', Menard Press, 2002.

SCHEME SPECIFIC RISKS	Public Sector	Private Sector
Provider fails to deliver facility by 1st April 2005		X
ISTC destabilises existing NHS services	X	
NCSC registration not obtained		X
Insufficient independent staff because of recruitment or registration difficulties		X
Insufficient NHS staff seconded by PB	X	X
PCTs fail to deliver work volumes – Demand Risk	X	X
Provider fails to meet quality and performance standards	X	
IM&T solution cannot conform to changing NPfIT* requirements	X	X
The Chain and Gaps inadequately resource the programme	X	
PROGRAMME SPECIFIC RISK		
Negative perception of ISTC – commercial failure if Patients and GPs do not choose to use it	X	

* National Programme for Information Technology
Source: East Lincolnshire NHS Primary Care Trust, Full Business Case for the Development of an Independent Sector Treatment Centre, April 2004, p. 32.

While a degree of risk-sharing is presented in the above matrix, in practice almost all risks were retained by the public sector.* Demand risk was in all cases assumed by the NHS under the 'Minimum Take' or 'Take or Pay' provision, guaranteeing the ISTC provider payment for all the procedures contracted for, and evidence was given to the Committee that this was happening in virtually all the Wave 1 contracts. Construction risk seemed to be allocated to the private sector. In the East Lincolnshire ISTC business case, for example, the risk of construction time over-runs was assigned to Capio (the preferred bidder for the chain of ISTCs in which the East Lincolnshire was one link). But when Capio failed to complete the construction of another ISTC in the chain on time, 'Oxfordshire PCT was forced to make a payment

*In PFI the principle has always been that risk is allocated to 'the party most able to bear it'. The implication of the way risk was assigned in the early ISTC business cases is that the providers were unable to bear risk (see Julie Froud, 'The PFI: risk, uncertainty and the state', in *Accounting Organisations and Society*, Vol. 28 (6), pp. 567-590, 2003)

of £1 million to Capio Healthcare UK, even though responsibility for building the Horton Treatment Centre in Banbury lay with the company...'.[94] Oxfordshire PCT was also unable to reclaim money prepaid to Capio for the procedures that were not in fact provided because the centre opened late.

Other risks nominally assigned to ISTC providers were also mitigated in practice. The risk of not being able to recruit enough staff under the additionality rule was largely mitigated in Wave 1 by the staff waivers and structural secondments discussed earlier; and for Phase 2 ISTC contracts it is mitigated by the abandonment of the additionality rule for all but a restricted list of occupations in the NHS, and its dilution even for the latter. The risk that registration with the National Care Standards Commission might not be obtained for staff brought in from overseas was mitigated by 'fast-tracking' (as we noted earlier, Netcare even believed that the responsibility for establishing the competence of its surgeons at Haslar lay with Portsmouth Hospitals NHS Trust); and the resultant increase in the risk that 'provider fails to meet quality and performance standards' was assigned to the NHS and borne by the Clinical Negligence Scheme for Trusts (and NHS patients).

The last of these risks – clinical risk – was tempered by the fact, which was inherent in the concept of specialist stand-alone centres, not integrated with a general hospital – that ISTCs were free to reject patients with more than one co-morbidity. This was presumably taken into account for VFM purposes in the calculation of the NHS Equivalent Cost cited above ('restrictions on the type of patient that can be admitted'). But it was often overlooked in other contexts relevant to VFM. Especially overlooked was the fact that the case-mix left for NHS trusts was higher-risk and so more expensive – a point made forcefully to the Committee by NHS clinicians.* Nothing in the DH presentation to the Com-

*Mr Ribeiro, the president of the Royal College of Surgeons, said: 'We use a grading, the American Society of Anaesthesiology grading, to determine how sick a patient is and we have very good evidence that a significant number of ASA 1 and 2 low grades have gone, leaving behind a lot of ASA 3 grades to be done, which are clearly more technically difficult and therefore are not good training opportunities'. See also the evidence from Mr Kelly, for the Royal College of Ophthalmologists, and Dr Peter Simpson, president of the Royal College of Anaesthetists (HC Report Vol III Ev 13-25).

mittee suggests that this featured in the calculation of the NHS Equivalent Cost.

But even when only relatively healthy patients are treated there is a risk that clinical errors may harm patients and lead to claims for damages; and given that ISTCs represented the first time that 'core' NHS secondary care services were being entrusted to private providers on a regular basis, it was obviously important. Yet at first it does not seem to have been clear whether this risk was really borne by the private sector. Early ISTC business cases are vague regarding the transfer of clinical risk to the private sector. Those we have seen suggest that 'clinical performance risk' was retained by the public sector.

In July 2004, however, the Clinical Negligence Scheme for Trusts (CNST) was officially extended to cover all ISTCs. The NHS Litigation Authority (NHSLA) said: 'We have agreed a special arrangement with the Department of Health whereby cover for clinical negligence suffered by NHS patients is afforded by the CNST. We are unable under the Statutory Instruments that govern the CNST to indemnify private companies direct. However, the way in which cover is organised is via the Primary Care Trust which refers the patient to the ISTC. This arrangement will pick up most patients who are referred to the private sector by the NHS'.[95]

Action Against Medical Accidents (AvMA – formerly the Association of Victims of Medical Accidents), however, were dissatisfied with this: 'No regulation or statute governs the indemnity position where the NHS contracts its services to another private sector company. Therefore contrary to the statement that "this arrangement [with ISTCs] will pick up most patients who are referred to the private sector by the NHS" – this is not the case'.[96] The AvMA still see the arrangements as unclear. In their evidence to the Health Committee the Association stated:

Many problems are now becoming apparent since the inception of ISTCs two years ago. We suspect that even more difficulties will surface as time goes on. Many of our lawyer members are reporting incidents where complications have arisen, particularly with patients demonstrating co-morbidities. The troubling feature has been that when something has gone wrong, no-one seems to accept the blame – each party pointing the finger at another...[97]

If true, this may have been because the document announcing the extension of the CNST to ISTCs was only released in January 2006 and not widely known about. As late as July 2005, for instance, the management consultancy Operis appears also not to have known about it (or it may simply have shared the scepticism of the AvMA), as it ran a seminar for investors in ISTCs focussing on clinical risk; nor was the extension of CNST to ISTCs mentioned to the Health Committee in 2006.

It is also unclear whether ISTCs are contractually required to contribute anything to the CNST. The ISTC Manual identifies the CNST as a risk-pooling scheme of which all PCTs and Acute Trusts are members, and 'In return for an annual contribution, members of the CNST are indemnified against damages and out-of-court payments which may be awarded to NHS patients and/or their dependants in the event of negligent care or treatment'. While private providers are not allowed to be members of the CNST in their own right, protection is afforded to them via a contractual indemnity from referring PCTs. 'As the PCTs are themselves protected by the indemnity afforded by the CNST', the Manual continues, 'they are in a position to hold the Provider [the private company] harmless against claims by NHS patients'. While ISTC contracts require compliance with relevant risk management standards, and specify the actions the company must take when faced with a patient claim, 'Providers are not required to make contributions to the CNST'. However, 'the Provider *may be* required to contribute to a Sponsor PCT's contribution if its claims history is worse than the NHS average for a comparable case mix' (emphasis added).[98] While the NHSLA document, 'Independent Sector Treatment Centres (ISTCs) and CNST', states that 'PCTs will not be subsidising providers', the same document also notes that 'There are several factors which contribute to the NHSLA's assessment of the additional contribution which each PCT will need to make to the CNST fund',[99] notably the types of procedure offered and their associated risk. Although the NHSLA claim that no public subsidy is involved, the documents would appear to indicate otherwise: that private providers are given indemnity cover for clinical negligence through NHS funds, to which PCTs and Acute Trusts will need to make additional contributions on the companies' behalf, and to which the companies may or may not be required to contribute, even if they have a bad claims record.

Some indication of the practical allocation of clinical accountability in ISTC contracts can be illustrated by some examples drawn from Michelmores' experience of NHS patients treated by Netcare at the Royal Hospital Haslar in Gosport, Hampshire. A Plymouth NHS patient was left with a third degree burn and suffered a dislocated hip following an operation by Netcare at Haslar during the company's initial 6-month contract from October 2003 to March 2004. After several meetings between Netcare and Plymouth Hospitals Trust to establish responsibility for both clinical negligence and surgical repair, an NHS consultant was assigned to do the repair work at a Nuffield hospital. While Netcare paid for the repair, the NHS paid the subsequent £40,000 indemnity to the patient.[100] Another hip operation at Netcare's ISTC at Haslar during the same period left an NHS patient with one leg shorter than the other and in such pain as to be unable to return to work for many months. The day he returned to work he dislocated his hip and was rushed to an NHS hospital by ambulance. The NHS paid for both repair and indemnity, again £40,000.

Following the extension of Netcare's contract at Haslar, a further claim of clinical negligence was brought against both the company and its sub-contractor, Medic Air, which had provided transport for a patient from Plymouth to Gosport. The NHS patient was at Haslar in November 2004 to have an arthroscopy on his left knee and the removal of a cyst on his right knee.. On waking from anaesthesia he discovered that surgeons had performed arthroscopies on both knees. During the subsequent journey back to Plymouth – some 200 miles – the ambulance driver stopped at a service station and the patient was invited out. He was on crutches and, due to the driver's failure to assist him, he stumbled and fell. Later the ambulance driver explained that she wasn't qualified to help him because she was only driving the ambulance for extra cash. Her main job was working for Plymouth aquarium.*[101]

It would appear from these examples that the issue of which party held clinical risk was not properly established in early ISTC contracts. Once problems began to occur the DH stepped in, and even backdated the extension of the CNST to cover ISTCs, so that the NHS would accept responsibility for cases of clinical negligence in ISTCs prior to July 2004.

In relation to VFM, what should concern us is whether the prices paid for ISTC contracts signed after the CNST was extended to cover ISTCs fell correspondingly. Given the blanket of secrecy covering the contracts, one can only speculate, but if investors in ISTCs originally assumed that it was necessary to insure against clinical risk, the cost of doing so must have been a significant element in the price. As the Michelmores cases show, the risk of serious claims for clinical negligence quickly manifested itself in some ISTCs. The fact that the NHSLA later claimed that 'significant savings' were made as a result of extending the CNST to ISTCs indicates that the original contract prices included provision for the cost of insuring against clinical negligence claims, but it declined to say how much the savings were, nor do we know who enjoyed the benefit of the savings.[102]

In the end what is most striking about the role of risk in the VFM analysis for ISTCs, as far as the evidence goes, is that not

*Medic Air, which Netcare had subcontracted to provide transport, has been the subject of enquiries by ambulance unions/organizations for advertising themselves as offering trained paramedical services. In February 2006 the BBC reported that 'Medic Air European, based at Crownhill Fort in Plymouth, called itself a "paramedic" service, but had no paramedics among its staff. It said they were employed on an "ad hoc" basis'. (Marcus Wraight, 'Private ambulance regulation call', BBC News, 11 July 2006, http://news.bbc.co.uk/1/hi/england/devon/5159406.stm.)

only was it all really borne by the NHS, but that the business cases we have seen do not refer to the risk of clinical negligence lawsuits, but do refer to the political risk that the public and GPs would turn against the whole programme – the 'negative perception of ISTC: commercial failure if patients and GPs do not choose to use it'. This risk, we may surmise, has a lot to do with the ambiguities and prevarications in the government's responses to the Health Committee, which clearly irritated its members (to the point where one of them remarked, 'We're wasting our time, chaps').[103]

Assisting reconfiguration

We noted earlier that at their final evidence session with the DH the HC 'were told of another objective for the ISTC scheme: to assist reconfiguration; for example, existing hospitals might be closed and some of the facilities replaced by an ISTC'.[104] This referred to a response by Ken Anderson, the Commercial Director of the DH, to a question about West Herts Hospital Trust, whose chief executive had told the Committee that they did not want the ISTC that the NIT had sought to impose on them in Wave 1 because the loss of demand would mean demolishing a well-functioning NHS hospital. Anderson replied:

> The flip side of that is that health economies* used the independent sector treatment programme as a reconfiguration tool as well. There is capacity in the NHS that we pay for that is not necessarily applicable to today's type of health care. Those are very detailed conversations around an extremely sensitive and extremely involved strategic issue for health economies…. it takes a detailed conversation with the health economy around what does reconfiguration look like and what does 21st century healthcare look like.[105]

---

*The expression 'local health economy' has been increasingly used by the DH and others to refer to all the bodies purchasing and providing NHS services, and the expenditures involved, in a given locality, usually the area covered by a Strategic Health Authority.

This was evidently an allusion to the idea, repeatedly revived but mostly not acted on over the years, of shifting some secondary health care out of hospitals, which account for half of the total NHS budget, into what are assumed will be less expensive 'community-based' settings. The decision, already mentioned, to drop seven of the 22 Phase 2 ISTCs originally proposed, and replace them with 'seven regional diagnostic schemes', covering the whole of England, was connected to this. In the shape of CATS (Clinical Assessment and Treatment Services) or ICATS (Integrated Clinical Assessment and Treatment Services) these Phase 2 independent sector operations were to vet GP referrals and divert patients from specialist treatment in hospitals to care in the CATS or ICATS centre itself, or some other non-hospital setting. This would put the private owners of these centres at the heart of NHS policy.

But nothing further was said about these to the Committee, which did not enquire about them, or feature them in its report. Instead it said that the decision 'to maintain a commitment to spend £550 million per year [on Phase 2] despite changing circumstances [the dropping of seven schemes] has not been explained, and seems to sit uncomfortably with the Secretary of State's admission that "in other [areas] it has become clear that the level of capacity required by the local NHS does not justify new ISTC schemes"'.[106] 'It is not clear', they added, 'whether this represents a failure coherently to articulate the situation or a more profound incoherence in terms of policy as opposed to presentation'.[107]

Conclusion

Yet this was to ignore something the Committee had confronted quite clearly at the beginning of their report: 'The Department', they said there, 'has referred to two main and distinct purposes, which have often and misleadingly been conflated: to increase the surgical capacity available to the NHS; and to involve the independent sector in an increasingly mixed health economy with all the benefits the Department claims this will bring'.[108] But the

Committee's conclusion shied away from deciding which was the true driving purpose. They said Wave 1 was 'not a carefully thought-out venture', and Phase 2 seemed to them to be more of the same. They called on the National Audit Office to investigate the 'wider benefits and costs' of the ISTC programme, 'in particular the extent to which the challenge of ISTCs has led to higher productivity in the NHS'.[109]

Perhaps this was a coded way of saying that the wider aims of the programme should be investigated and disclosed; but there were more than enough clues in the evidence available to the committee to show that the programme was no leap in the dark, but on the contrary the crucial first step in a fairly well thought-out plan to create a private provider industry in the UK to compete with the NHS using NHS funds, and eventually to subject all health care to market principles. The Committee either failed to see this clearly, or chose not to focus on it.

The result was a report which expressed scepticism or disquiet about the series of particular claims made for the ISTC programme by the government, but refrained from commenting on the rather obvious fact that its main aim, which Professor Appleby had pointed out to them, lay elsewhere. It observed that ISTCs had not made a 'major direct contribution' to increasing capacity and that it was 'far from obvious' that ISTCs were needed in all the areas where they had been built. It thought ISTCs had increased choice, but in the absence of information on clinical quality, did not offer an informed choice. They were not 'necessarily more efficient' than NHS Treatment Centres, nor was there any evidence that they were driving innovation in the NHS. The Committee thought the 'threat of competition' might have had a 'significant effect' on the NHS, and criticised the DH for not ensuring that any such effects were assessed or quantified.[110] It also criticised the DH for not collecting data on outcomes that could be compared with NHS data, but did not demand that it do so forthwith, and dismissed as 'strident and alarmist' and 'anecdotal' the criticisms they had heard from clinicians of clinical standards in ISTCs. They saw the lack of integration of ISTCs into the

NHS as a weakness, and called for it to be improved. They said they had been denied the information needed to judge whether the ISTC programme would destabilise the NHS, but did not enter a protest at this. But in spite of this fairly comprehensive list of failings, and the fact that its value for money could not be assessed, the Committee did not say that the ISTC programme should be scrapped.

In retrospect the most remarkable aspect of the Committee's work is not only that it failed to discuss the wider aim of the ISTC programme, although it had been pointed out to them, and was even acknowledged at the outset of their report; but also that the 'independent sector' at the heart of the programme – the corporations concerned, their corporate histories and aims, the links between them, their shared vision of the future healthcare market that would eventually replace the existing NHS – did not feature in it all. No questions were put to the Commercial Director about the kind of commerce he was bringing into the NHS, or the logic of the dynamic it was hoped and expected that it would develop, or what implications this might have for the founding principles of the NHS.

The aim of Chapter 3 of this book is to try to make the real function of the ISTC programme clear by partially remedying this omission, and looking at the role of the programme in promoting the government's ultimate aim of creating a healthcare market.

Notes

1   House of Commons Health Committee, *Independent Sector Treatment Centres*, Fourth Report of Session 2005-06, Vol III, Ev. 51.
2   The Secretary of State in HC Report, Vol III, Ev. 86.
3   HC Report, Vol. I, para. 26.
4   Ibid.
5   Freedom of Information response from Wendy Lipsidge, Contact Centre Team, The Information Centre for health and social care, Query reference number 69446.
6   Personal communication from the DH Data Collection, Validation & Analysis Team, 18 July 2007.

7   Personal communication, Central Contract Management Unit, Department of Health, 6 July 2007.
8   HC Report, Vol II, Ev. 1.
9   FOI Response from the Department of Health, DE00000205646, 30 April 2007.
10   FOI Response from the Department of Health, DE00000241293, 22 October 2007.
11   Ibid.
12   Ibid.
13   Healthcare Commission, *Independent sector treatment centres: a review of the quality of care*, July 2007, p. 6.
14   HC Report, Vol I, para. 36.
15   HC Report, Vol I, para. 29.
16   HC Report, Vol III, Ev. 2.
17   HC Report, Vol I, para. 35.
18   HC Report, Vol I, para. 132.
19   HC Report, Vol II, Ev. 62-166
20   HC Report, Vol III, Ev.. 61
21   NHS Employers, 'ISTCs, Human Resources Framework', January 2005.
22   Cited in the Unison document 'Operating for Profits', September 2005. We have so far been unable to obtain a copy of this document, although its existence and the point made have been corroborated in telephone discussion with Andrea Hester, Head of Programmes, NHS Employers, 12 October 2007.
23, Melanie Newman, 'Empty wards and promises', *Hospital Doctor* 5 October 2006.
24   Sam Lister, 'Pioneering hospital could be mothballed for lack of patients' *Times,* 14 February 2005.
25   'Hospitals to "fatten up" NHS centre', *Hospital Doctor,* 2 March 2006.
26   Seamus Ward, 'Running on Empty', *Public Finance,* 3 December 2004.
27   Melanie Newman, 'Empty wards and promises', *Hospital Doctor,* 5 October 2006.
28   Ibid.
29   Ibid.
30   HC Report, Vol I, para. 35.
31   HC Report, Vol III, Ev. 16.
32   HC Report, Vol II, Ev 99.
33   HC Report, Vol III, Ev. 63.
34   HC Report, Vol I, para. 139.

35   HC Report, Vol I, para. 121.

36   'DH looking for "more innovation" from second wave ISTCs', *Healthcare Market News*, October 2005.

37   HC Report, Vol I, para. 45.

38   HC Report, Vol I, para. 48.

39   Department of Health, *Treatment Centres: Delivering Faster, Quality Care and Choice for NHS Patients*, January 2005.

40   Department of Health, press release, 2 February 2005.

41   John Williams, 'Faster, better - and still free. Scaremongers dismiss NHS reforms as creeping privatisation. In fact, the private sector will refresh the service's core values'. *Guardian* 27 May 2005.

42   Nick Astbury, 'Medical evidence on outsourcing', *Guardian*, 30 June 2005.

43   George Osborne, 'Speech by the shadow chancellor to the Policy Exchange thinktank', *Guardian Unlimited*, 17 July 2006.

44   Department of Health, Ken Anderson, *Commercial Director. Independent sector treatment centres*, 16 February 2006.

45   'ISTC medical director left over quality issue', *Hospital Doctor*, 26 May 2005. The article added that 'Dr Verma and one other ophthalmologist together performed more than half of the 10,000 cataract operations carried out in the mobile units last year'.

46   National Centre for Health Outcomes Development. *Preliminary Overview Report for Schemes GSUP1C, OC123, LP4 and LP5*, 3 October 2005.

47   HC Report, Vol III, Ev. 48.

48   NCHOD, *Preliminary Overview*.

49   HC Report, Vol III, Ev. 49

50   NCHOD *Preliminary Overview*, p. 5, Section 3.1.3.

51   Department of Health. *Preliminary audit of Independent Sector Treatment Centre schemes heartening – Warner*, 11/11/2005.

52   Healthcare Commission, *Independent Sector Treatment Centres: A review of the quality of care*, July 2007, p. 7.

53   Ibid, p. 7.

54   Ibid, p 24.

55   Ibid, p. 25.

56   Ibid, p. 15.

57   Ibid, p. 32.

58   Ibid, p. 9.

59   'ISTCs to usher in a new breed of doctor?', *Healthcare Market News*, November 2003.

60   HC Report, Vol I, para. 63.

61   British Medical Association. '*Impact of Treatment Centres on the*

Local Health Economy in England', December 2005.
62 Ibid.
63 Sarah Boseley. 'NHS forced to fix bungled private sector hip replacement operations', *Guardian*, 10 March 2006.
64 Ibid.
65 Angus Wallace. *'ISTCs:* How the NHS is left to pick up the pieces', *BMJ*, 11 March 2006.
66 Sarah Boseley. *Guardian*, 10 March 2006.
67 Melanie Newman, 'Audit shows ISTC failures', *Hospital Doctor*, 20 April 2006.
68 Kelly SP, Mathews D, Mathews J, Vail A, 'Reflective consideration of postoperative endophthalmitis as a quality marker', *Eye*, Vol 1, 1-8, 2005.
69 Ferris JD, 'Independent sector treatment centres (ISTCS): early experience from an ophthalmology perspective', *Eye*, Vol 19, 1090-1098, 2005.
70 Verita, Hampshire and Isle of Wight Strategic Health Authority, 'An investigation into the events surrounding the early revision of hip prostheses amongst patients operated on between 10 and 20 November 2003, as part of a contract with Netcare Healthcare UK Limited', 21 October 2005. www.hiow.nhs.uk/ha-05-134.pdf
71 HC Report, Vol I, para. 72.
72 HC Report, Vol I, para. 73.
73 HC Report, Vol II, Ev. 2-3.
74 Kings Fund: *'Public Views on Choice in Health and Healthcare'*, October 2005.
75 HC Report, Vol I, para. 41.
76 John Carvel, 'GPs offered payments to send patients private', *Guardian*, May 11 2006; Melanie Newman, 'Practices get £130 per referral to ISTC', *Hospital Doctor*, October 26 2006.
77 HC Report, Vol II, Ev 166.
78 HC Report, III, Ev. 58.
79 HC Report, Vol III, Ev. 60.
80 Ibid.
81 Department of Health, *Growing Capacity: A new role for external providers in England*, June 2002, p. 5.
82 See John Reid, 'No, it's not privatisation', *Guardian*, September 12, 2003: Department of Health 'Speedier surgery for thousands of patients', *Press Release*, 12 January 2004; and Department of Health. *Treatment Centres: Delivering Faster, Quality Care and Choice for NHS Patients*, January 2005.
83 HC Report, Vol II, Ev. 4.

84 HC Report, Vol I, para. 38.
85 HC Report, Vol III, Ev 8.
86 HC Report Vol III, Q 9 and HC Report Vol I, para 39.
87 See Ken Anderson's oral evidence to the HC, HC Report, Vol III, Ev. 7, col. 2.
88 HC Report, Vol I, para. 103.
89 HC Report, Vol I, para. 103; HC Report, Vol III, Ev. 110.
90 'Private Corporations in the NHS', BBC Radio 4, File on Four, 17 October 2006, http://news.bbc.co.uk/1/shared/bsp/hi/pdfs/02_10_06_fo4_nhs.pdf.
91 HC Report, Vol III, Ev. 146-47.
92 HC Report, Vol III, Ev. 87.
93 HC Report, Vol III, Ev. 147.
94 Melanie Newman, 'PCT billed £1m for ISTC delay', *Hospital Doctor*, 11 January 2007.
95 Cited in the evidence submitted to the Health Committee by Action against Medical Accidents (AvMA), HC Report, Vol II.
96 Ibid.
97 HC Report, Vol II, Ev. 37.
98 ISTC Manual, p. 24.
99 NHS Litigation Authority, 'Independent Sector Treatment Centres (ISTCs) and CNST', http://www.nhsla.com/NR/rdonlyres/79E694BA-A4AB-45A4-95B8-E0A7499DCB99/0?ISTCsfactsheet.doc. January 2006.
100 http://medneg.michelmores.com/netcare/orthopaedic-page2.asp
101 'Plymouth man suffers "botched" operation and is then injured again during ambulance journey home', Michelmores Press Release, 12 July 2006; 'Private ambulance regulation call', BBC News, 11 July 2006, http://news.bbc.co.uk/1/hi/england/devon/5159406.stm
102 NHS Litigation Authority 'Independent Sector Treatment Centres (ISTCs) and CNST', January 2006, p2; and personal communication from the NHSLA, 15 October 2006.
103 Mr David Amess, HC Report, Vol III, Ev. 106.
104 HC Report, Vol I, para. 26.
105 HC Report, Vol III, Ev. 104-05.
106 HC Report, Vol I, para. 139.
107 Ibid.
108 HC Report, Vol I, para. 13.
109 HC Report, Vol I, para. 108.
110 HC Report, Vol I, para. 56.

CHAPTER 3: THE ISTC PROGRAMME IN CONTEXT – CREATING A HEALTHCARE MARKET

The true significance of the ISTC programme can only be grasped by seeing it as a crucial step in the replacement of the NHS as an integrated public service by a healthcare market, in which private providers will play a steadily increasing role. This means focusing on the DH's leading role in creating a market, in close collaboration with private providers, while seeking to minimise the risk that the public, who are strongly supportive of the NHS and have never been invited to vote for its dismemberment, will react against the strategy and bring it to a halt.

The ISTC programme is central to the strategy for two main reasons. First, the strategy implies that a growing number of NHS doctors and nurses will be employed by private healthcare companies. Because the main official rationale for creating ISTCs was to add to elective capacity, ISTCs had to rely initially on recruiting most of their clinical staff from outside the NHS, but with the additionality rule effectively abandoned for Phase 2, staff transfers to ISTCs will become increasingly common. Seconded and part-time work by NHS staff will gradually give way to careers in private companies. While still on a small scale, relative to the elective and diagnostic case-load of the whole NHS, ISTCs are playing a crucial role in normalising this idea.

Second, the favourable terms given to Wave 1 ISTCs showed the established domestic private healthcare providers that they had to restructure, away from high-cost provision of services to a limited clientele of privately-insured patients, and join the competition for NHS patients, which they have rapidly done. This has resulted in an England-wide network (the 'Extended Choice Network') of private hospitals and clinics able to compete with

NHS trusts for NHS patients – officially at NHS tariff prices, and not only for elective care.

Several parallel processes of restructuring in the NHS itself are closely linked to the ISTC programme. Securing public acquiescence in the introduction of private providers into all parts of the NHS is a continuing concern. For this reason the boundary between NHS and private treatment centres (ISTCs) has been blurred. On the one hand ISTCs have been renamed 'NHS' treatment centres, to emphasise that they are now, in the words of the DH, 'firmly part of the NHS family';[1] and on the other hand a strong market orientation has been developed for the remaining publicly-owned NHS centres through, for example, encouraging the formation of doctors' 'chambers' (on the lines of barristers' chambers) and the payment of fee-for-service bonuses to surgical teams.

Closely related to this is the drive to 'reconfigure' secondary care by moving elements of it, especially the treatment of chronic diseases, into non-hospital settings, in which private providers can be expected to find profitable niches – something CATS are explicitly designed to promote – alongside the introduction of private companies to undertake commissioning of both primary and secondary care for PCTs.

As secondary care is thus 'unbundled' and parcelled out to ISTCs and other new and old private providers, the role of consultants, hitherto firmly based in NHS hospital trusts, becomes crucial. The negotiation of a new consultants contract, leading to both pressures and encouragement for consultants to form independent chambers and offer their services to the highest bidders, public or private, is also a significant stage in the process of market formation.

And governing the whole process is the need to manage risk – the risk that the full implications of market creation will become apparent to a public far from convinced that companies working to maximise shareholder value will improve universal access to the highest quality of health care, and that as a result the programme will ultimately be abandoned. The need to manage this risk accounts for the level of official secrecy, information management and dissimulation that is such a marked feature of the ISTC programme.

In this Part we briefly outline each of these dimensions, starting with the government's aim – which was clearly outlined in 2000-2002, though subsequently downplayed – of creating a healthcare market.

ISTCs and the creation of a market

In concluding that the ISTC programme was 'ill thought-out' the Health Committee was being unfair to the Department of Health. Numerous statements in White Papers, guidance documents and prospectuses, from the *NHS Plan* onwards, stress a commitment to 'diversity' and 'pluralism' of provision. The underlying rationale was to secure efficiency in the NHS by exposing it to competition. The goal was made particularly clear in the June 2002 document already cited, *Growing Capacity: A new role for external providers in England,* which announced 'the creation of a new sector in health care provision in England' which would be 'additional to existing publicly-owned NHS provision'; the NHS would 'be the core business of units in this sector' and these units would be 'set up and run by run by independent operators'. The aim was 'to bring new entrants… into the health care market'.[2] Even this formulation, however, obscured the real nature of the project – to spend a growing share of the NHS budget on private, for-profit providers, and to shift a growing proportion of the NHS workforce into them.

The ISTC programme was a response to the problem that the UK's existing private health sector could not provide the kind of competition the DH's strategy called for. Accounting for only 14 per cent of all healthcare spending (about half the OECD average), it offered high-cost treatment to a small market of privately-insured patients, and relied almost exclusively on NHS clinicians working part-time. Moreover its main competitive advantage over the NHS – cutting out waiting time for elective care – was being eliminated by the increased funding going to the NHS after 2000, which was steadily reducing waiting times for NHS patients. The DH needed, therefore, to engineer the formation of a new kind of private healthcare provider, offering low-cost, high-volume treatments at prices competitive with those of NHS trusts. The obvious way to begin was to separate out certain standardised, low-risk clinical activities, or segments of such activities, with low infrastructural costs relative to turnover – and offer them to new providers on highly attractive terms. This could be presented as adding extra capacity to help meet the government's targets for reducing waiting times for diagnoses and elective treatments. The result would be to create a model that the domestic ('incumbent') private providers would be forced to follow, and a precedent for diverting a growing portion of the NHS budget to the private sector generally.

The scale requirements of the new private market

The strategy was adopted in 2002 and the first ISTC opened in October 2003. The question then was how fast and how far it needed to be developed. The Commercial Directorate commissioned an 'IS-TC Market Sustainability Analysis' (MSA), which was presented to Health Ministers in June 2004, 'to help inform thinking in preparation for the next phase of independent sector (IS) procurement'. A copy with some key sections omitted was obtained by the *Guardia*n through a Freedom of Information request in February 2005.[3]

The MSA defined its purpose as providing 'a commercial view and supporting analysis to take into consideration when defining the scope of the next waves of procurement of the Independent Sector Treatment Centre (ISTC) programme'. Its scope was 'to evaluate the current and future market sustainability of the IST market'.

With the introduction of six new players, the ISTC programme has begun to establish a new market in the UK... The ISTC programme is driving a dramatic shift in private provision. We now have the beginnings of a "mid-tier market" where independent sector providers have entered the UK based on a high-throughput, low-cost business model where the NHS is the primary customer.[4]

But with only the volumes of work currently contracted for with the ISTC sector in 2003-04, and the number of market competitors in the sector, the report predicted that within 4-7 years the market was likely to 'stagnate and ultimately collapse'. Instead, the authors said, 'We assume that the DH wants to create a whole new pluralistic market, one that provides the following outcomes: competitive pricing is maintained across all regions of the country; ISTC choice is available to every patient; a market is established that is able to deliver up to 15% of the total NHS demand...' But, it added, 'market growth opportunities are extremely important if it [the emerging market] is to be able to access capital at reasonable costs and meet investor expectations...' And 'the only drivers which new providers will use to decide whether to have a presence in the UK IST market is if the volume of business in the market is attractive enough to justify dedicating a strong management team and giving high priority to this business...'.[5]

The MSA report concluded that the Wave 1 providers already operating, or shortly due to start, would need 'at least 200,000 additional procedures per year to sustain the transformation of their business model whilst using their workforce and infrastructure capacity'. But to go beyond this and create a sustainable 'whole new pluralistic market', with '3-4 national providers with ~120k+ procedures each, plus 4-6 regional or specialist providers with ~90k procedures each... [and] transformation of other parts of [the] secondary care market, high patient choice, creating real competition to NHS monopoly', the market needed 'to grow by at least 450k additional procedures per year'.*[6]

*The context makes it clear that this actually meant 450,000 a year on top of the 234,000 a year the MSA report expected to be provided by Wave 1, i.e. a total of 700,000. The totals suggested for a 'whole new pluralistic market' seem to vary a good deal from one part of the report to another, although this may be partly an impression caused by the omission of sections of parts of the report in the published version on grounds of commercial confidentiality.

The scale of Phase 2 makes sense in this context. The number of additional elective procedures expected in Phase 2 was, as we saw in Chapter 1, about 400,000 a year (ISTCs and the Extended Choice Network combined); Phase 2 also included an additional 1.5 million diagnostic procedures a year.[7] On top of this, in September 2006 the then Secretary of State, Patricia Hewitt, stated that there would be no ceiling on the amount of private sector work carried out on behalf of the NHS.[8] Government policy was thus aiming at a market even larger than that which the MSA saw as being necessary in order to make it secure.

The ISTC programme must therefore to be seen in the context of the goal of market sustainability that the DH was pursuing. Market sustainability calls for market growth to a level of service volume sufficiently attractive to private providers. Locally-defined needs are secondary. Once this is grasped, much that the Health Committee said it found puzzling becomes clear enough. The reason why the DH committed itself to spend the full £3 billion on Phase 2 elective ISTCs, in spite of having accepted that there was no need for seven out of the 22 additional ISTCs originally planned, was that the market required this level of spending to be sustainable.* Other ways of spending the money on private providers would be found, especially in the shape of CATS or other new kinds of agency.

---

*According to the *Financial Times* of 8 November 2005, 'The decision to commission another 250,000 operations a year from the private sector, and to buy in several hundred million pounds a year of diagnostics, has settled an internal argument within the Department of Health. One side argued that the health service needed more operations from the private sector to hit its waiting time targets. The other said it was only more diagnostic capacity that was needed, to shorten "hidden waits": the time between seeing a doctor and getting the tests needed for a clear diagnosis. The answer was to have both. What that will provide, according to Ken Anderson, the NHS commercial director, is a sustainable NHS market for the private sector that will still be attractive once the initial contracts for the first wave of independent treatment centres run out in five years' time'. (Nicholas Timmins, 'Private sector set to gain access to "sustainable NHS market"', *Financial Times*, November 9, 2004.)

Restructuring the private sector and the Extended Choice Network (ECN)

As Laing & Buisson noted, 'the UK's established private health-care providers were dealt a blow' when Wave 1 [ISTC] contracts were predominantly given to overseas companies and new entrants.[9] The fact that the established domestic providers, particularly BUPA, Nuffield and the General Healthcare Group (GHG), missed out on the lucrative early ISTC contracts prompted them to restructure their businesses in time for the next wave of procurement. In the short term the G-Supp contracts gave them a taste of what was on offer, and the chance to put in place the new forms of organization required. The impact of the ISTC programme in driving this restructuring was dramatic. As Ken Anderson told the Health Committee,

> When we first started the [ISTC] programme probably the biggest change before any ISTC even had planning permission was the change in the incumbent private sector. BUPA reorganised completely and sold 12 hospitals; BMI streamed its business into two halves, one addressing specifically the NHS and the other taking care of their private patient base, and Capio, which is owned by a Swedish company, did a lot of changes and became more efficient...[10]

In June 2004 BUPA invested £100m in a modernization plan for its remaining hospitals to 'standardize business and clinical procedures in a bid to bring customer prices down' and 'to accommodate contracts in G-Supp and ISTCs'. [11] In June 2006 BUPA was named preferred bidder for two ISTCs in the north-east and northwest of England, for 5,000 and 6,000 procedures a year respectively, and in August 2006 for 105,000 diagnostic procedures in the southeast. This was the restructuring which permitted the DH for the first time to place bulk (G-Supp) contracts with BUPA, and also made it possible for BUPA to start bidding successfully for Phase 2 ISTC contracts.

In February 2004 Nuffield bought out Vanguard Healthcare, which on a sub-contractual basis provided mobile units to Netcare for cataract operations. In May 2004 Nuffield also won one of the largest G-Supp contracts made with an established private provider, to deliver 17,000 procedures for 20 Strategic Health Authorities at a price of £40m; and in June 2005 it gained its second G-Supp contract, in tandem with BUPA and GHG, to carry out 5,000 general surgery procedures at 18 of its hospitals. The proportion of NHS patients treated in Nuffield's hospitals grew from 6.3% in 2003 to nearly 20% in 2005.[12] In March 2007 Nuffield announced that its Plymouth Hospital had begun offering services through the Extended Choice Network,[13] a list of private hospitals which NHS patients were entitled to choose and which were willing and able to treat NHS patients at NHS standards and at the NHS tariff discussed below. By August 2007 157 hospitals were listed in the ECN.[14] As the MSA had predicted, a shift to high-throughput, low cost modelling in elective care had stimulated 'increased market intensity and cost pressures at all levels'.[15]

GHG (General Healthcare Group) responded to the challenge by selling up: in the largest ever healthcare deal in Europe, and the biggest globally in over a decade, GHG was sold to the South African healthcare conglomerate Netcare, strongly active in Wave 1 ISTC contracts, for £2.2bn. The buyout retained both divisions of GHG's business: its portfolio of 50 BMI private hospitals with 2400 beds, and Amicus Healthcare, which tendered for NHS contracts. This merger pointed to the prospect of a wider range of NHS work being carried out by the private sector, including general and perhaps even emergency surgery. Netcare's Chief Executive Mark Adams said that in South Africa the company ran 400-600 bed district general hospital-style institutions that include A&E Departments. 'Aspirationally we'd like to run hospitals in the same way as we do in South Africa. But we don't expect to be given a chance to do that until we have proved that we can do a good job with the contracts currently on offer'. [16] Mark Smith, the Chief Executive of Netcare's rival Mercury, said Netcare's aspiration was 'not unrealistic. I can see that happening in 5-10 years. Things are changing so fast it would not surprise me to see private companies invited to manage acute trusts in that time'.[17]

Meanwhile, however, a new and indefinitely expandable element was being quietly added into the ISTC programme – the so-called Extended Choice Network (ECN) of independent providers. It was first mentioned in May 2005, in Patricia Hewitt's opening speech as Secretary of State for Health, in which she outlined plans for a 'massive' increase in private sector procurement.[18] The DH was said to be estimating 'a procurement value of £150m - £200m, suggesting that it anticipates an additional 75,000 to 100,000 finished consultant episodes a year under the scheme'.[19]

Unlike ISTCs, providers in the ECN would not be guaranteed any minimum levels of income or activity, and PCTs would only pay for work that was actually carried out. But a 'rough' element of guaranteed work seemed to be implied by the fact that ECN contracts would 'take the form of "call off" contracts... prenegotiated by baselining activity against a rough volume'. What was evidently involved here was the need to adjust the supply of private clinical provision, at a price close to the NHS tariff, to the demand for private provision that the government's plans for 'patient choice' was intended to produce. The industry source just quoted summed it up as follows:

> It is expected that providers will begin delivering procedures under the initiative from April next year [2006] at the same time all foundation trusts and ISTCs are due to be included on patient choice menus. At the moment, it is not clear whether the ECN will be the only route for providers wishing to be included in the choose and book system, but the DH said the initiative was a forerunner for 2008, when patients will be able to choose any provider, NHS or independent sector, that meets NHS standards and the prices the NHS is prepared to pay.[20]

Confidential documents shown to the private health industry in March 2006 said that under the ECN, providers would not have to show that they could provide substantial levels of performance or commit to minimum volumes of activity. They would just have to have IT systems which were compliant with the government's computerised 'choose and book' system.[21] Moreover a much wider range of procedures would be included in the ECN than in the ISTCs of Wave 1 and Phase 2. Only emergency and cosmetic surgery procedures were excluded.

A month later the documents – 'Choice at Referral: Guidance framework for 2006/7' – were produced by the DH publicly. [22] All Foundation Trusts, ISTCs and approved IS providers would be automatically members of the ECN and could 'add services to the national menu' (i.e. to the list of treatments which NHS patients could choose to get from non-NHS providers). While FTs could add services to the menu immediately, ISTCs would initially only be able to put on the menu activities covered by their current contracts. But they could apply to add other treatments, and PCTs were 'strongly encouraged to add IS providers selected in this way to their local menus'. Services on the menu would be provided at the NHS tariff.

The ECN was officially launched in May 2006. In August it was reported that the Department of Health had 'signed a deal worth £200m with 14 independent healthcare companies', intended to 'deliver an additional 150,000 procedures per year, on an "ad hoc" basis, as part of the DH's second wave of elective care private sector procurement'. The companies would be 'added immediately to the central extended choice menu, which currently consists of all foundation trusts and some independent treatment centres'. BMI Healthcare, (part of the Netcare group), was the biggest winner, securing 44 contracts across the country. Other contract winners included BUPA, Nuffield, Capio, Centres for Clinical Excellence, Mercury Health, and Nations Healthcare. Several small private companies were 'also understood to have won small contracts to provide local services to NHS patients'.[23] Each contract would run for 5 years. Although the DH had told

the Health Committee in March 2006 that the ECN would operate 'on an ad hoc basis', determined by patient choice, it quickly
became clear, as *The Times* noted, that the DH had 'opted for
centralised bulk buying to give the NHS more advantageous
terms'. [24] Or to put it another way, only by being offered more or
less guaranteed volumes of work would private providers be willing to offer treatments at or near the NHS tariff price. The same
article also noted that the procurement was undertaken 'without
any fanfare':

> The contracts were not announced last week by the Health
> Department, prompting suspicions among health service
> professionals that the Government did not wish to high-
> light the move before the TUC and Labour conferences,
> where private sector provision remains controversial. But
> the department suggested yesterday that there was nothing
> unusual about an announcement not having been made. A
> spokesman said: "This is not a new procurement but part
> of the second wave of procurement from the independent
> sector which was launched in May last year".

Industry commentators thought that with the addition of the
ECN the independent sector could be performing 680,000 elective operations on NHS patients in 2008, and perhaps many
more – worth perhaps 40 per cent or more of its total activity
– if 'patient choice' led to a 'mass migration' of NHS patients to
independent providers. Most of the major providers, they noted,
had 'already positioned themselves to take advantage of the potential increase in NHS activity, albeit at reduced margins, and
are included on the ECN. Insurers have also begun to respond to
the threat of an improved NHS by developing cheaper and more
innovative products…' [25]

The ECN is thus a framework within which a steadily growing transfer of elective services to the independent or corporate
sector is expected to take place. Why it should be described as
part of the ISTC programme is not obvious, unless it is because

corporate providers needed to be assured that the balance of the £5.6 billion committed to the ISTC programme, which is now not going to be spent on new ISTCs, will be devoted to the ECN, providing a measure of security during the transition to a much larger market.

Restructuring the NHS

1) The assimilation of NHS TCs to ISTCs – 'NHS Elect'

As already mentioned, by 2007 ISTCs had been authorised to call themselves 'NHS Treatment Centres' and had been admitted as full members of the NHS Confederation, the NHS managers' association. At the same time the already established NHS Treatment Centres (NHS TCs) were being reshaped on increasingly market principles, led by 'NHS Elect'. This was initially an association of a handful of NHS TCs, but quickly became a private company, funded by the DH with subscriptions from the NHS TCs which belonged to it. Starting in 2002 with three affiliated NHS TCs, NHS Elect now has 29 members and an active set of full-time executive directors. According to the DH, NHS Elect 'began as a "First Movers" programme to pioneer new ways of working in NHS TCs in 2002/2003… It is essential that the programme provided by NHS Elect is seen in the context of a wider programme of reform and that the TCs within this group are pilot sites for innovation, change and policy development'. [26]

While the language of NHS Elect is usually couched in vague abstractions such as 'innovative care pathways' and 'optimizing patient outcomes through sharing best practice', what is most significant about it for present purposes is its role in introducing private-sector forms of organization (doctors' chambers, and partnerships or joint ventures with IS providers) and payment mechanisms (fee-for-service), and the wider dissemination of these models within NHS Treatment Centres, most of which were soon affiliated to it. By 2005 the organisation was promoting a number of 'chambers' schemes. One of its directors, Jim Timpson, had a 'special interest in the Independent Sector' and had 'worked with member trusts on treatment centre transfers, es-

tablished a Chambers Support programme for consultants working in independent partnerships and forged links between NHS
treatment centres and major insurers'.[27]

NHS Elect was working with two groups of surgeons on this
basis. One was a team of orthopaedic surgeons in southwest London and the other was the Consultant Eye Surgeons Partnership,
which had nine groups of ophthalmic surgeons in London, Newcastle, Bristol, Surrey and other parts of the country. Both were
bidding for contracts to provide operations for NHS patients
in both NHS-run and private treatment centres. Andy Black, a
former NHS manager who now acts as a management consultant, said the developments were a 'logical outcome of the supplier market in healthcare the government is creating. One of the
more radical options being explored, though not yet tried, would
involve groups of surgeons and anaesthetists quitting the NHS to
provide an entire service such as orthopaedics or eye surgery back
to the NHS on contract'.[28]

A related 'first mover' mechanism also promoted by NHS
Elect was 'fee-for-service' (FFS) contracts: 'a new model of care
in which surgeons and anaesthetists are paid a fee for each procedure rather than a salary. Individual NHS doctors and nurses
can pocket bonus payments worth hundreds of pounds for carrying out extra operations'.[29] This seems to be an overstatement:
the fees in question appear to be bonuses on top of salary, not
a substitute for salary. 'The radical new fee-for-service scheme
could see clinical teams divide up bonuses of £250 a session for
treating more than a benchmark number of patients, while nurse
specialists could take home £400 a month bonuses on top of their
pay for exceeding a target number of cases, as a variety of pilot
schemes are set up at 32 NHS trusts'.[30] In July 2004 pilot schemes
were announced, building on the NHS Elect model. The pilots
involved 400 doctors and other clinical staff and set a target of
8,000 additional operations and 6,000 outpatient consultations.

In December 2004 the FFS Pilot Programme was reviewed for
the DH by the private sector consultancy Serco Health. Its report
said the DH was using FFS arrangements 'to incentivise consult-

ants and other NHS staff to deliver NHS activity'. A degree of diversity between schemes was identified: in some pilots, clinical teams received a fixed sum of money for each additional operation completed, while in others bonuses were paid to whole teams and the funding was used to purchase extra equipment. However all had 'in common an activity-based reward for quantified target outcomes', which are 'heavily influenced and/or directly affected by current developments in the NHS including: waiting time reduction (and its impact on private practice), Payment by Results, Patient Choice, Agenda for Change* and the new consultant contract'.[31]

The review highlighted a number of problems: there needed to be 'careful consideration [of FFS arrangements as a form of incentivization] in the context of extensive literature on incentives and performance related pay which identifies opportunities and risks'. FFS in healthcare in particular required 'careful consideration in the context of international experience which is largely cautionary'; quantitative evaluation of the pilots was problematic owing to the largely informal and unstructured conduct of the programme; and the objectivity of the evaluation was also compromised in various ways .The review concluded: 'The pilot programme demonstrated that FFS as a form of incentivization can facilitate change and promote desirable outcomes but not without difficulties and risks which must be carefully managed'.[32]

Yet less than two months later, in February 2005, the DH announced that the FFS programme was to be 'rolled out' on a larger scale.[33] The then Health Minister John Hutton said 'Hospitals participating in the scheme are using Fee for Service to help transform the way patient care is delivered, improve efficiency and create extra capacity. The scheme covers a range of treatments, including orthopaedics, ophthalmology and general surgery...The initial evaluation of the pilots shows that the new ways of working have made a significant impact in helping reduce waiting times...'[34]

---

*A programme of terms-of-service reform which covers all NHS staff groups apart from doctors, dentists and very senior managers.

2) 'Reconfiguration'

By 2006 the argument that ISTCs were primarily about increasing capacity had worn thin and was replaced as a leading theme by the idea that the District General Hospital (DGH) was an outdated form of service delivery for secondary care. ISTCs were trailblazers for this, and the corporate owners of ISTCs were in the forefront of a new call for reconfiguration. Lord Darzi's plan, Healthcare for London, is the most publicised example to date.*[35] Based on what are presented as technological and public health arguments, the plan argues that health care in London should be reorganised on seven different levels – the home ('more healthcare should be provided at home'), polyclinics (offering a wider range of services than a general practice), 'local' hospitals, 'major acute' hospitals, specialist hospitals, and 'academic health science centres' (to be 'centres of clinical research excellence'). Evidence of the proved superiority of these ideas is not included in the report. But the various costs involved taken together 'would combine to create a massive affordability gap that can only be bridged', Lord Darzi told *Health Investor*, 'if the NHS works with its partners... in the voluntary and private sector'. This was confirmed in October 2007 by the new Secretary of State, Alan Johnson: 'After months of mixed messages on the issue, Mr Johnson said the independent sector would be involved in providing 150 new health centres and 100 new GP practices'.[36]

A significant force driving these ideas seems to be the National Leadership Network for Health and Social Care (NLN). Established in December 2004 to replace the NHS Modernisation Board (which had been given the task of pushing through the process of reform outlined by the *NHS Plan*), the NLN said, in a report for ministers which was leaked to the press in March 2006, that all acute hospitals, but especially smaller ones, 'face "irresistible" pressure for change from more competition in the provision of NHS care... and the ability to shift more care out

---

*Lord Darzi's interim report *Our NHS Our Future: NHS Next Stage Review* (Department of Health, October 2007), setting out a '10-year vision for the NHS', is less specific, though based on the same concerns as his report for London.

of hospital'.[37] Some hospitals, it said, will remain principal providers of care but will have to subcontract various elements of
care, subject to periodic contestability. New employment models
were needed across the evolving networks of hospital and community services which 'would "remove key clinical staff from the
direct employment of individual hospitals", instead employing
them through new over-arching organisations'. Such organisations could include 'independent sector companies, ones run by
"social enterprises", or NHS staff leaving direct employment and
forming "chambers"'.[38]

The chambers model was already being pursued by BMI
Healthcare, now Netcare's private patient hospital chain in the
UK, which had 38 doctors chambers groups 'operating from its
hospitals', and was said to be in discussion with a further 90.[39]
Another example was Centres of Clinical Excellence, a company
founded in October 2005, with private equity backing, by a group
of former employees of the investment bank Goldman Sachs. In
July 2007 the new company bought three ISTCs from Nations
Healthcare. It claimed to have 745 consultants as co-owners or
partners, and was planning to open a chain of private hospitals
and specialist clinics, treating both private and NHS patients.[40]

All these ideas implied, of course, that in commissioning secondary care PCTs would increasingly 'unbundle' care into separable
packages and parcel it out to the new range of private providers
on offer. A consultation document, *Commissioning framework for
health and well-being*, was published by the DH in March 2007,
which stresses the value of a wide range of smaller providers and
calls on commissioners to 'actively encourage a strong provider
market, based on a diverse supply community from all sectors'.[41]
A report was also commissioned which mapped the 'third sector'
with a view to contracting more NHS work from organisations in
it.[42] The best known of these organisations are non-profit 'social
enterprises', including those expected to be formed by community care personnel, hitherto directly employed by PCTs, to compete for contracts with private companies. But the third sector is
also key to reconfiguration in the sense of moving more work out

of hospitals. In Suffolk, for example, a group of GPs and consultants formed Suffolk Healthcare Ltd to bid for a contract to provide all outpatient work in ENT, as 'they feared the PCT could award the work to an international healthcare company using overseas doctors'.[43] Whether Suffolk Healthcare Ltd will prove able to survive competition from large commercial providers in the longer run remains to be seen.

Thus all elements of the NHS (barring perhaps major teaching hospitals (or 'academic health science centres') are being increasingly fragmented into marketable items, adapted to the resources and interests of a variety of new market entrants. The government also signed a 'framework contract' to help enable primary care trusts to employ the private sector in commissioning. The 14 contractors include four big US health insurers and care managers, Aetna, Humana, Health Dialog Services and UnitedHealth, as well as UK health specialists such as Bupa, Axa PPP and Tribal, and the consulting firms KPMG and McKinsey'.[44] If Strategic Health Authorities expect or even require PCTs to make use of them, these companies seem likely to play an important role in facilitating the insertion of private providers into the emerging range of secondary care options.

3) *CATS*

A parallel facilitating role seemed to be implicit in the establishment of Clinical Assessment and Treatment Centres (CATS), which emerged as a significant component of Phase 2 of the ISTC programme. In 2007 it became apparent that negotiations over Phase 2 of the ISTC programme were not proving easy. By July the number of centres under negotiation was down to ten, instead of the 22 originally envisaged. Negotiations for two, accounting for a third of the total number of procedures under negotiation in January, had been abandoned.* Gradually shifting demand risk to the providers, as anticipated by Patricia Hewitt

---

*These were the South London 'CASS' contract for which Clinicenta was the preferred bidder, with an annual planned total of 299,000 procedures a year, and the West Midland contract, for 29,000 procedures from which the preferred bidder, Nuffield, withdrew, citing delays in finalizing the contract. See Table 3 in Part 1.

for Phase 2 – 'tapering' the proportion of procedures covered by 'Take or Pay' – was said to be a significant difficulty. There was even speculation that the new Brown government might be abandoning the ISTC policy.[45] What seemed more likely was that Wave 1 had already accomplished the government's key objective of initiating the break-up of NHS secondary care and restructuring the private sector to take over more and more of it. A new wave of private sector provision could be rationalised in terms of the reconfiguration agenda, which CATS would facilitate.

In mid-2006 plans were announced to set up seven 'Integrated Clinical Assessment and Treatment Service' (ICATS, later renamed just CATS) operations in Greater Manchester. There were two joint preferred bidders: Netcare, and Partnership Health Group in partnership with Alliance Medical. ICATS differed from ISTCs in that their function was not just to treat patients referred to them by GPs, but first to vet GP referrals with a view to diverting patients away from hospitals for treatment either in the ICATS themselves, or in some other specialist centre; or to send them back to be treated by GPs or other forms of community-based care.

That this was part of a wider strategy became clear when in September 2006 the British Association of Dermatologists found that over half of 102 'clinical leads' who responded to a survey reported that their local PCTs were setting up CATS schemes, which they expected to 'divert away' up to half their departments' patients.[46] Then, in early 2007, it was announced that PCTs in Cumbria and Lancashire would in future send all patients referred by GPs to one of seven Clinical Assessment, Treatment and Support Services or CATS (sometimes also called 'Capture Assess and Treat Services'), with Netcare again as the preferred bidder. The bid was to include the provision of treatment in six specialties – orthopaedics, rheumatology, ENT, general surgery, gynaecology and urology.[47] According to *Hospital Doctor*, 'Central Lancashire PCT has already decided that 100% of GP referrals in all the specialties except urology will be sent to the CATS centre for "paper triage"'.[48] In Bolton it was announced that 'around 90 per cent of

GP referrals would be handled' by the new private centres.[49]

At the time of writing no reference to CATS or ICATS was to be found on the DH website,* but it seems reasonable to assume that this new kind of centre was what the DH was referring to when it told the Health Committee that Phase 2 would have the further objective of 'assisting reconfiguration'. This time there is no hiding the fact that local hospital finances will be destabilised, since the objective is precisely to contract or close some hospital services, or indeed whole hospitals, while the private sector provides many if not most of the alternative services. The implication is clear that many NHS staff will lose their jobs and have to find work instead with the private operators of CATS and ICATS, or other private providers. Official comments by local trust managers have been about 'minimising' job losses, not avoiding them.[50]

As before, hospital consultants complained that they had not been consulted.[51] As before, central procurement (which the DH had told the Health Committee would give way to local procurement in Phase 2) made local opinion something to be assuaged, not listened to. The contracts had already been centrally negotiated. For example Ian Cumming, chief executive of North Lancashire PCT, told a meeting of the Independent Sector Commissioning Board (ISCB) in Kendal, Cumbria: 'We were not able to consult on whether using the independent sector to run CATS is a good idea or not. It is Department of Health policy and the principles of CATS and use of the independent sector is already determined'.[52] And when a public consultation was forced on the DH by local opposition, the chief executive of North Lancashire PCT said it would 'not include the decision to offer the services to Netcare'.[53] Choice also seemed once again to be reduced, rather than increased, since patients would only have a choice of hospital if a CATS centre judged them suitable to be sent for treatment at a hospital.

---

* A Department of Health FOI response to a request for an explanation of the various CATS/ICATS acronyms can be found in the Appendix.

4) *The consultants contract*

Since the government's aim was that the private sector's share of NHS clinical work should grow without limit, and the ISTC programme (with the training of junior doctors included as an option in Phase 2) was the private sector's entering wedge, consultants were crucial to it, as they also were to the new Extended Choice Network of private hospitals treating NHS patients that was being created alongside the NHS hospital system. This made the negotiation of a new consultants contract as important for secondary care as the new GP contract and Alternative Provider of Medical Services contracts had been for the privatisation of primary care.[54] Negotiations on a new contract – the first since 1948 – began in 2002, just as the ISTC programme was being launched. The government said its aim was 'to introduce a stronger unambiguous contractual framework with greater management control, in return for a career structure and pay system rewarding those consultants who made a long term commitment to the NHS and the biggest contribution to service delivery and improving health services'.[55]

At first sight this seemed to be inconsistent with the aim, announced in the *NHS Plan,* of moving 'away from a centrally-controlled state system and towards a more devolved model in which a variety of different organizations provide services' (as a Kings Fund report put it).[56] On closer inspection, however, the two ideas might be seen as strategically linked. The new contract proposed by the government threatened consultants with tighter managerial control within the NHS. The reaction against this on the part of a majority of consultants in England was predictable, and it coincided with the expansion, in England, of opportunities within the private sector. The way the negotiations were conducted by the DH suggests that the government may have had the tacit, or perhaps alternative, aim of bringing about a greater willingness on the part of some consultants to change to working in chambers outside NHS salaried employment, offering their services to private as well as NHS providers at competitive rates, or even taking up full-time employment with private providers.

A key element in the contract proposed by the government was that newly-qualified consultants should be banned from undertaking private practice for seven years. This was comprehensively rejected. The BMA's lead negotiator pointed to the obvious contradiction: 'At a time when the Secretary of State is encouraging more NHS patients to be treated in the private sector, such a ban would be illogical, unworkable and probably illegal'.[57] Of course, if the government's aim was to encourage a growing number of consultants to work more or less full time in the private sector, a ban would not be so illogical, separating those who wanted to stay from those willing to move.

The government, however, gave up the proposed ban and improved the remuneration package on offer. But the consultants still voted to reject the package. The decisive factor was hostility to increased managerial control and the target-based culture associated with it, and the proposed linking of pay rises to performance targets set out in agreed job plans. There was also hostility to the way the government was seen as having conducted the negotiations, threatening to impose a contract, and holding out the prospect of purely local variants.

Consultants in Scotland and Northern Ireland voted by small majorities to accept the contract. It was in England and Wales, where alternative employment in the private sector was beginning to look like offering a serious alternative career, that consultants voted 2:1 against acceptance. Eventually, in November 2003, the consultants voted 3:2 (in the UK as a whole) to accept a much-modified version of the contract. The main remaining element of enhanced managerial control was a provision that consultants must work one extra NHS session of 4 hours in addition to the basic working week of 40 hours before they are able to undertake private work without prejudicing their NHS pay progression. It left many consultants feeling their autonomy and willingness to work had been compromised. A survey by *Hospital Doctor* found that only 23% of hospital doctors said they were prepared to stay in the NHS until 65; the rest said they were planning to retire early, change career, do more private work or move abroad. Thirty per cent said they planned to leave and establish private practice chambers.[58]

The reference to 'chambers' in this connection can be illuminated by looking at a commentary on the consultants contract story by Dr Penny Dash. Dr Dash was now a freelance health policy consultant, but she had been Head of Strategy and Planning at the DH from 1999 to 2001, when the *NHS Plan* was produced. Her article was written in November 2002, just after the consultants had rejected the first contract.

In it she speculated that the no-vote might have 'played into the hands of Messrs Blair and Milburn', adding: 'Yesterday's resounding rejection of the new consultant contract could have positive and far reaching implications for the way NHS care is delivered - not least because it may open the door to more private sector provision of healthcare'. While representing the no-vote as 'a blow to the Government', she suggested that 'Messrs Milburn and Blair usually have a back-up plan. This "Plan B" may be to tacitly encourage far-reaching changes which may offer the only hope of reducing waiting lists and developing a truly "patient centred" healthcare service'.[59]

Dr Dash suggested that

Ministers may want to encourage surgeons, and indeed other groups of doctors, to form their own companies (or join existing private health providers) to sell their services back into the NHS. Consultants, in this case it would be mainly those involved in routine elective surgery, may see this as a chance to make more money, and free themselves from NHS bureaucracy:

1)   Ophthalmologists could form their own companies and negotiate with the NHS to perform cataract removals, sometimes performed in private hospitals, sometimes in under-used NHS operating theatres.
2)   Groups of orthopaedic surgeons could resign from the local hospital trust and provide hip replacements services

on a private contractor basis.

3)   Pathologists could form a start-up business, which will be able to raise capital to invest in much-needed technology to improve quality of care and substantially increase treatment throughput.

4)   Radiologists could join forces with suppliers of X ray machines and scanners to provide a "full service solution" to ailing NHS hospitals.

Freed from the 'stifling grip' of the NHS (and the Treasury),

> private surgical provider companies [which would later be called "chambers", on the lines of barristers' partnerships] could more easily invest capital in new equipment, use IT to its full potential and develop innovative new ways of working. As competing organisations (rather than in-house monopolies) they would have to be better employers in order to recruit and retain the best staff; they would be driven to implement efficient working practices, develop true customer service, and ensure and demonstrate high quality clinical care.

Dr Dash's enthusiastic presentation of private chambers models, juxtaposed with her reference to the 'stifling bureaucracy' of an increasingly target-oriented, monolithic NHS, is suggestive. It was the *NHS Plan*, of which she had been one of the authors, which had launched the target-driven productivity culture referred to. While it is impossible to know whether the government's aim in seeking to tie consultants more closely to the NHS was consciously aimed at achieving the opposite, it certainly conflicted with its aim of market creation, and may have served the latter aim better in the end. The established relationship between the NHS and its consultant workforce notoriously contained ambiguities and trade-offs, including having the right to private practice, balanced against doing extensive unpaid work for the NHS. At the heart of the relationship, however, was the consultants' longstanding insistence on autonomy; yet this was what the proposed new contract explicitly proposed to reduce. Perhaps Plan B was in fact Plan A all along.

Yet voting against the contract entailed a risk. Outside the contract consultants would have to learn to compete, and competition would eventually force down their incomes. As private providers restructured in order to compete with NHS trusts, they would not be able to pay consultants the high fees they had commanded up to now for part-time work treating privately-insured patients. It was 'rumoured in the private health care industry' that the new NHS contracts of Phase 2 ISTCs and ECN providers implied consultant fees as much as 50% below BUPA insurance rates.[60]

Consultants were in any case already facing downward pressures on their fees for treating privately-insured patients. The insurers faced a loss of premium income as patients found that NHS waiting times had fallen, and as 'patient choice' allowed them to choose to be treated as NHS patients by private hospitals in the Extended Choice Network. Led by BUPA, which had 40 per cent of the private medical insurance market, the insurance companies now asked consultants to accept significantly lower fees per operation in return for being offered a higher volume of private work. After an initial retreat in face of resistance from ophthalmologists, BUPA created a new 'network' of approved hospitals, i.e. a list from which most of its insured 'members' would have to choose. Although initially limited to cataract treatments, this approach was widely expected to become general. BUPA Insurance's medical director, Dr. N-J Macdonald, said, 'Doctors have to recognise that unless changes are made, there will not be any private practice'.[61] The BMA and the Federation of Independent Practitioners Organisations saw it as the beginning of managed care on the lines of American HMOs, and it seems likely that they were right.[62]

Managing and mitigating political risk

The political risk was real that public opinion would eventually grasp the full significance of ISTCs, and the market strategy they were spearheading, before the new private providers had consolidated and become entrenched inside the NHS. The risk is evident in the underperformance of Wave 1 ISTCs, insofar as this has been due to the reluctance of patients to be referred to them, or of GPs to refer to them. It is also evident in the delays in finalising contracts for the elective part of Phase 2. Phase 2 was supposed to become operational in 2007, but by August 2007 only two contracts had been signed,[63] and in November a further six schemes were abandoned, including the two most strongly opposed CATS schemes, leaving only eight elective and two diagnostics schemes still under negotiation.[64] Many aspects of the way the programme was introduced reflect the constant need to mitigate the political risk. Here we indicate just three of the most obvious mechanisms involved.

1) The 'policy community'

The various mechanisms through which the long-term aims behind the ISTC programme are being achieved have their own logic and also reflect the market forces – the efforts of the companies and their lobbyists – that are increasingly at work in reshaping health provision on market lines. But they are all facilitated by an inner cadre of people with shared ideas and inside knowledge, operating with unprecedented facility across the public-private boundary; a cadre which gradually expands as a wider circle of NHS managers and clinicians are confronted with the new project and start adapting to it. The 'policy community' of health policy-makers, management consultants, healthcare company executives and market-oriented think-tanks, operates largely out of the public eye.

Within the NHS, the National Leadership Network mentioned above was established because, the DH says, 'the next phase of reform requires a new leadership model and change management process'.[65] The NLN 'brings together 150 people who have a major contribution to make in steering the next phase: patients and users of services, clinicians and managers, professional leaders, inspectors and regulators and leaders from partner organisations', and 'will provide collective leadership for the next phase of transformation, advise Ministers on developing policies, ensure rapid feedback from the front line and promote shared values and behaviours'.[66] What exactly these shared values and behaviours are is not knowable; the Network's webpage says, '**This is not a public website**. Access is restricted to members of the National Leadership Network'.[67] Publications, resources and contacts are all password-protected.

At the summit of the health 'policy community' the boundary between the public and the private sector has become increasingly indistinct. As we have already noted, Ken Anderson came to the Commercial Directorate from the private sector, and returned to it at the end of 2006. Tom Mann, a senior civil servant who as head of the DH's National Implementation Team had been responsible for negotiating Wave 1 ISTCs, left to set up a consultancy and then became Chief Executive of Capio Healthcare UK, the ISTC provider which won one of the major 'spine' chains. Simon Stevens, health adviser to the Prime Minister and one of the main authors of the *NHS Plan*, left to become president of UnitedHealth Europe, which is closely involved in the privatisation of primary care. Alan Milburn, a former Secretary of State for Health, became an adviser to Bridgeport Capital, the parent of Alliance Medical. Penelope Dash, Head of Strategy and Planning in the DH when the *NHS Plan* was written, worked for Kaiser Permanente and the Boston Consulting Group and joined the board of Monitor, the foundation trust regulator. Darren Murphy, a former special adviser to the Prime Minister, and previously special adviser to the Secretary of State for Health, became director of corporate lobbyists APCO UK in September 2005. APCO's clients include nearly all the Wave 1 and Phase 2 ISTC companies, and these companies have subsequently formed an 'NHS Partners Network', which bills itself as 'a loose alliance of independent healthcare organisations which provide diagnosis, treatment and care for NHS patients'.*[68] By 2007 the Commercial Directorate had a staff of 190, of whom just eight were civil servants, the other 182 being recruited from the private sector.**[69]

The work of this policy community becomes easier as each new element in the matrix exercises its own pressure on adjacent ones. The healthcare market regulator Monitor, for example, recently put Foundation Trusts on notice that they must identify the services and treatments on which they make a profit, and be prepared if necessary to abandon those on which they make a loss. Bill Moyes, the chairman of Monitor, said Foundation Trusts should find out which treatments they provided were profitable, and consider expanding them, and which were not; these they should if necessary give up 'and let someone else do it'; '… the time may come when Foundation Trusts may be able to walk away from a service, provided we are confident that the primary care trust has alternative suppliers'.[70] Given that many if not most PCTs will not have two competing Foundation Trust providers nearby, this

*The NHS Partners Network comprises Alliance Medical Limited; Amicus Healthcare (part of General Healthcare Group); BUPA Hospitals Ltd; Capio Healthcare UK; Clinicenta Ltd; Mercury Health; Nations Healthcare Ltd; Netcare Healthcare UK Ltd; Nuffield Hospitals; Partnership Health Group; UKSH Ltd. One of Murphy's first coups in his new role was establishing a meeting between the Partners Network and the Prime Minister: 'The most significant independent providers of diagnosis and treatment services for NHS patients announced today the formation of a new network with a commitment to the long-term success of the NHS. The NHS Partners Network is being launched at a press conference in Westminster, following a meeting with the Prime Minister in Downing Street to discuss how its members are helping to deliver improved services and outcomes for NHS patients'. ('NHS Partners Network launched', Netcare website, 19 Feb 2006, http://www.netcareuk.com/netcare/media/news/index.jsp?ref=4&year=2006)

**Some months after the appointment of Channing Wheeler, a former senior executive at the US healthcare corporation, UnitedHealth, as the new Director General of the DH's Commercial Directorate, the *Health Service Journal* reported that 'In the run-up to this [the appointment of Mr Wheeler] *HSJ* interviewed a number of former senior staff about life at the commercial directorate, what it achieved, the times when it had failed and just why it is so controversial. They range from one man who left because, as he put it, "I could not stomach the ethics of what I saw going on around me", to the man who says "as a taxpayer, and never mind personally, I was never unhappy with anything we did"'. The question of the number of 'interim' staff recruited on a day-rate basis from the private sector concerned several respondents. 'It is not just the numbers that cause concern. Critics of the Directorate point out the close links between top-level interims, many of whom worked with Mr Anderson [the former Director General] at Amey [a company heavily involved in PFI contracts]. They point to multi-million pound contracts awarded to companies that have interims on [Commercial Directorate] project teams'. (Daloni Carlisle, 'Controversial and divisive: Whitehall's own Big Brother', *HSJ*, 28 June 2007.)

primarily means private suppliers.

Another straw in the wind was a statement by Ken Anderson, who had left the Commercial Directorate to join the Swiss bank UBS in November 2006. Two months later, in January 2007, he mused publicly that

> the days when the NHS can choose which services it puts out to tender are coming to an end... European commercial law was set to force the NHS to open up many more of its services to bids from private sector companies... My personal conviction is that once you open up NHS services to competition, the ability to shut that down or call it back passes out of your hands... At some point European law will take over and prevail... In my opinion we are at that stage now. [71]

The more private sector providers had invested, the more this investment increased 'almost exponentially the likelihood that they will challenge in the courts procurements that they feel do not follow appropriate procurement law'. Of course a future government could decide to commission all future health care from public providers and overcome any potential legal obstacles at the EU level. But it seemed likely that Anderson's views reflected the prevailing thinking of the policy community in which he had recently played such a central role.

2) *Information control and presentation*

An adequate public understanding of any of the key features of Wave 1 could well have jeopardised it: the scale of the public subsidy; the almost complete absence of risk transfer; the *de facto* deduction from NHS capacity; the destabilisation of NHS trust finances, leading to deficits, service closures and job cuts; and the lack of publicly-reported clinical audit. For this reason information about the programme had to be kept to a minimum. No routine data are published on it. Such information as the government has released has been in response to the Health Committee enquiry, parliamentary questions and FOI requests. Data on the quality of clinical work have not yet been published in a form that can be compared with those of NHS providers. The only quantitative data supplied are numbers of procedures. But 'procedures' are not defined, and the sources of the figures given are not provided. In the data given to the Healthcare Commission, very large numbers of primary care procedures suddenly appeared, without explanation, for the year 2006-2007 (see Table 4). Plans for the programme are similarly opaque.* Financial data are denied because it is said that to reveal them would breach commercial confidence, or prejudice the government's future efforts to secure best value. As a result the ISTC programme is, as one member of the Health Committee told the Commons, 'an evidence-free policy zone'.[72]

A few health journalists are broadly aware of what is happening, but by and large the handing over of NHS functions and staff to the private sector is able to proceed without the public fully realising it. The full range and speed of the marketisation programme is known and understood only by a relatively small circle of people who meet regularly in settings such as Laing and Buisson's annual Acute Healthcare conferences, with health ministers in attendance.

3) 'Integration'

The government has been greatly helped by the way the threat to NHS funds and staff has been framed by the medical profession. The keyword here is 'integration'. As the private sector share of NHS funding expanded, NHS doctors and surgeons reacted by calling for private provision to be better 'integrated' with NHS provision. It was a constant refrain in the evidence given to the

---

*In August negotiations were reported as 'ongoing' for an ISTC for Bedfordhsire and Hertfordshire that had not been mentioned in January. Negotiations were also said to be ongoing for 'Cumbria and Lancashire CATS', while financial close was said to be 'expected shortly' for 'Cumbria and Lancashire Electives', not mentioned as a separate project in January. The feeling one gets is that since the negotiations are confidential no great importance is attached to reporting them accurately (see Department of Health, 'Phase 2 Electives and Diagnostics Update', version 2, 9 January 2007; and response to an FOI request of 3 August 2007 from the Customer Service Centre, Department of Health).

Health Committee by both NHS consultants and ISTC representatives. The rationale was that it was necessary for continuity of patient care (especially in case of complications), and for the best use of resources. The Health Committee noted that 'witnesses thought it important that ISTCs were physically close to facilities which could support both integration in terms of staff and a full range of medical support'.[73] The Healthcare Commission opined that 'where there is greater integration between the ISTC and the local NHS, the local health economy – ... the local hospital and the local PCT – ... where you have it working integrally as part of that local healthcare economy, it all works very much better'.[74] The DH was happy to agree. It proposed that new ISTCs should be located in or next to NHS hospitals, that the additionality rule should be curtailed, and that NHS consultants should be used in ISTCs.[75]

The chairman of the BMA consultants' committee, Paul Miller, and his successor Jonathan Fielden, expressed anxiety about the scale of the transfer of resources to ISTCs, but in practice focussed on trying to ensure that NHS consultants were able to work in them. While publicly attacking ISTCs as dangerous to patients (Dr Miller told the 2005 BMA seniors conference that 'as things stand, I would not accept an MRI scan or elective surgery from these independent sector treatment centres'), the leadership resisted a motion opposing them, arguing instead that ISTCs could bring about 'a sustainable expansion of capacity' and that the rule excluding NHS consultants from working in them (i.e. the additionality rule) should be abolished.[76] A year later, commenting on the Health Committee's report, Miller was quoted as saying: 'For the last three years, the BMA has been shouting from the rooftops about its concerns regarding ISTCs. I am particularly pleased to see the Committee agrees that the Department of Health needs to go further in enabling NHS doctors to work and train in ISTCs, as I believe this will benefit standards and integration of patient care'.[77]

Conclusion

Central to the ISTC programme is the fact that it implies a substantial and growing transfer of staff from NHS to private sector employment. But thanks to the way the programme has been presented publicly, the implications have been largely ignored, even in the local press, except where significant job losses in local NHS trusts, or service closures, are threatened. The reality is that Wave 1 was primarily a bridgehead for the establishment of a new kind of private sector in NHS secondary care, allowing it to become 'normalised' as a provider of NHS care and initiating a process in which the distinction between public and for-profit provision becomes increasingly blurred.

Phase 2 will see this blurring spread throughout the NHS, as secondary care is 'unbundled' and the NHS budget is distributed among an expanding range of private providers. Additionality is no longer a barrier (and it may even be applied retrospectively to Wave 1, helping with the large backlog of procedures contracted for).[78] Staff will be available, because NHS hospital trusts are laying staff off, or not replacing them when they retire, since they are losing the funds that are going to ISTCs and the growing number of private and 'third sector' bodies bidding for parts of the services hitherto provided by hospitals – services now being unbundled and put out to tender by PCTs complying with the new commissioning regime. A draft DH workforce strategy document leaked to the press in January 2007 predicted a surplus of 3,200 NHS consultants by March 2011.[79]

So Phase 2 ISTCs and Extended Choice Network providers will be able to deliver, and subsequently expand, taking on surplus NHS consultants as they are laid off, or finish their training without NHS jobs to go to. Phase 2 contracts also include training options, so junior hospital doctors will be able to make the switch; the Royal Colleges have already signalled their approval. The BMA will try to protect their terms, but a major part of the point of shifting staff to private providers is to save money by changing the terms on which staff are employed. In his evidence

to the Health Committee the General Counsel of the Commercial
Directorate was very explicit about this:

> Strictly speaking, the Department's position is: No, there is
> no requirement to impose obligations on the private sector
> to engage any medical workforce on identical terms to the
> NHS... We have no visibility of the terms and conditions on
> which any staff engaged by the IS sector are employed...[80]

And in due course NHS trust terms will have to follow suit,
if they are to compete successfully with private providers whose
staff costs are significantly lower.

In June 2006 a forum of experts from the public and private
sectors organised by the King's Fund declared that the 'government must state unequivocally that it wants to create a healthcare market involving a range of different providers to ensure the
success of its ambitious health reforms'. The group's chairman
said: 'A supply-side market is being created in health care out of a
powerful mix of tariffs, incentives and new providers. This offers
tremendous opportunities but it also carries great risks'.[81] The
final part of this statement is crucial; and once it is recognised
it is easy to understand Ministers' reluctance to declare openly
their aim of market creation using NHS staff, patients and public money. The process does entail great political risk, which accounts for the secrecy in which it is conducted, and the elabo-
rate and wide-ranging measures to mitigate risk outlined above.
Indeed given the scale of public subsidy to both phases of the
ISTC programme it is likely that one of the largest risk-pricing
elements in the contracts was political risk; practically all other
risks had been retained by the public sector. In other words, the
public is paying for contracts, a major cost constituent of which
is the possibility that they will discover what the real aim of the
contracts is, and reject it.

Notes

1   *The Government's Response to the Health Committee's Report on Independent Sector Treatment Centres,* Cm 6930, October 2006, p. 1.

2   Department of Health, *Growing Capacity: A new role for external healthcare providers,* June 2002, p. 2.

3   Department of Health, 'Independent sector treatment centre (IS-TC) market sustainability analysis'. The redacted version of the report was on the DH website in February 2005, and was last updated on 8 February 2007. It consists of 12 un-numbered pages.

4   Ibid, section 2.

5   Ibid, sections 7, 2, 3 and 8.1.

6   Ibid, sections 2 and 7.

7   Department of Health, 'Phase 2 Electives and Diagnostics Update', January 2007.

8   John Carvel, 'Hewitt rules out limiting size of private sector role in NHS', *Guardian,* September 20 2006.

9   Laing & Buisson, 'British providers rocked by treatment centre snub', *Healthcare Market News,* October 2003.

10   HC Report, Vol III, Ev. 7.

11   Laing & Buisson, *Laing's Healthcare Market Review* 2006-2007.

12   Ibid.

13   Nuffield, 'Choice extends for NHS patients as Independent Provider goes live on ECN', 1 March 2007. http://www.nuffieldhospitals. org.uk/admupldfiles/Nuffield%20Hospital%20Plymouth%20live %20on%20ECN.pdf

14   Department of Health, Freedom of Information response DE00000228102, 13 August 2007.

15   Department of Health, 'Independent sector treatment centre (IS-TC) market sustainability analysis'.

16   Melanie Newman, 'Netcare eyes NHS acute hospitals', *Hospital Doctor,* 14 September 2006.

17   Nicholas Timmins, 'South Africans make £2.2bn GHG swoop', *Financial Times,* 26 April 2006.

18   'Huge increase in independent sector procurement as Hewitt ups pace of NHS reform', *Healthcare Market News,* June 2005.

19   Ibid.

20   Ibid.

21   'Smaller providers set to benefit from ECN contracts', *Healthcare Market News,* March 2006

22   Department of Health, 'Technical Notes for Choice at Referral

　　　– Guidance Framework for 2006/7, April 2006.

23　'14 private firms win place on choice menu in £200m deal', *Health Service Journal*, 31 August 2006.

24　Philip Webster, 'Clash expected on £200m private contracts for NHS', *The Times*, August 31, 2006.

25　'Orthopaedic procedures will act as test-bed for full NHS choice', *Healthcare Market News*, May 2007.

26　Department of Health website, NHS Elect: A summary of their work, Last modified date: 3 December 2004.

27　http://www.nhselect.nhs.uk/

28　Nicholas Timmins, 'Private treatment at risk, says BMA', *Financial Times*, 21 September 2005.

29　Tash Shifrin, 'Bonus plan to cut NHS waiting lists', *SocietyGuardian. co.uk*, July 9 2004.

30　Ibid.

31　Serco Health, 'Review of National Health Service "Fee For Service Programme"', December 2004.

32　Ibid,. p. 4

33　Department of Health, 'Bonus scheme to reward clinicians rolled out further across NHS', *Press release*, 15 February 2005.

34　Ibid.

35　NHS London, *Healthcare for London: A framework for action*, 2007.

36　'Backing for private sector's NHS role', *Financial Times*, 5 October 2007.

37　Nicholas Timmins, 'Doctors in "chambers" seen as option for reshaping NHS', *Financial Times*, March 14 2007.

38　Jimmy Burns and Nicholas Timmins, 'Health service needs radical restructuring, ministers told', *Financial Times*, March 22 2006.

39　*Healthcare Market News*, March 2006.

40　*Healthcare Market News* October 2005, April 2007 and July 2007.

41　Department of Health, *Commissioning framework for health and well-being*, March 2007, p. 42.

42　Department of Health, 'Third Sector Market Mapping', Research Report prepared for Department of Health by IFF, 3 February 2007.

43　*Doctor*, 13 February 2007

44　'Backing for private sector's NHS role', *Financial Times*, 5 October 2007.

45　E.g. 'Cabinet reshuffle: private sector fights to stay on agenda', *Health Service Journal*, 5 July 2007.

46　Melanie Newman, 'Dermatologists hit by referral management',

Hospital Doctor, 7 September 2006.

47   Ibid.

48   *Hospital Doctor,* 25 January 2007.

49   *Bolton News,* 22 January 2007.

50   For example: 'Pledge to keep hospital cuts to a minimum', *Bolton News,* 22 January 2007.

51   'Consultation on CATS a "sham", says BMA', *Healthcare Market News,* February 2007.

52   'CATS centre moves a step nearer', *Lancashire Evening Post,* 23 March 2007.

53   'Cumbria and Lancashire CATS contract goes to consultation', *Health Service Journal,* 23 November 2006.

54   For the effects of the new GP contract see Allyson M. Pollock, *NHS plc,* second edition, Verso, 2005, pp. 147-164 and 248-50; and Allyson M. Pollock and David Price, 'Privatising Primary Care', *British Journal of Medical Practice,* Vol, 56 (529), August 2006, pp. 565-66.

55   National Audit Office, 'Pay Modernization; A New Contract for NHS Consultants in England', 19 April, 2007.

56   'Designing the "new" NHS': Ideas to make a supplier market in health care work', *Kings Fund,* June 2006.

57   'Consultants oppose private practice ban', *Healthcare Market News,* March 2001.

58   'Stressed consultants eye NHS exit', *Healthcare Market News,* August 2003.

59   Penny Dash, 'Plan B on the consultant contract', *SocietyGuardian. co.uk,* November 1 2002.

60   'BUPA presses ahead with network launch', *Healthcare Market News,* April 2007.

61   Ibid.

62   *Healthcare Market News,* April and June 2007.

63   Freedom of Information response from the Department of Health, DE00000228102, 13 August 2007.

64   Department of Health press release, 'Ministerial statement by the Secretary of State', 15 November 2007.

65   Department of Health, 'Patricia Hewitt calls for NHS leaders to listen to patients to help improve family health services', 19 May 2005.

66   Department of Health, 'Creating a Patient-led NHS - Delivering the NHS Improvement Plan' Section 4.19, 17 March 2005.

67   http://www.nationalleadershipnetwork.org/public/default.aspx

68   NHS Partners Network: Launch of NHS Partners Network, February 16 2006. http://www.nhspartnersnetwork.com/press/press_16Feb2006.htm

69   'Private sector role in pioneering healthcare scheme to be slashed', *Financial Times,* 15November 2007.

70   Nicholas Timmins, 'Hospitals told to focus on profit centres', *Financial Times* 12 March 2007.

71   Nicholas Timmins, 'European law looms over NHS contracts', *Financial Times* 16 January 2007.

72   Charlotte Atkins MP, Commons Hansard, Column 157WH, 10 May 2007

73   HC Report, Vol I, para. 114.

74   HC Report, Vol III, Ev. 268.

75   HC Report, Vol I, para. 112.

76   Melanie Newman, 'BMA seniors split over use of private sector', *Hospital Doctor,* 16 June 2005.

77   BMA Response to the Independent Sector Treatment Centre Report, *UK Public Health News,* 6 August 2006.

78   Personal communication from Dr Tom Frusher, BMA Policy Analyst, 10 September 2007.

79   'NHS facing glut of consultants and nurse shortage', *Guardian,* 4 January 2007.

80   HC Report, Vol III, Ev. 106.

81   Nicholas Timmins (ed), 'Designing the "new" NHS: Ideas to make a supplier market in health care work', *Kings Fund,* June 2006.

POSTSCRIPT

Following Tony Blair's departure as Prime Minister in July 2007 early speculation pointed to the possibility of a reversal in the use of the private sector within the NHS. As the procurement process for Phase 2 of the ISTC programme became increasingly protracted, the *Financial Times* reported that the new Health Secretary, Alan Johnson, 'might cancel perhaps the bulk of the second wave of contracts that have yet to be signed for further ISTCs' in what might involve 'a significant policy shift'.[1] Launching a year-long review of the health service, Johnson stated that the reforms, and notably the ISTC programme, 'had come across as "ideologically driven"' and there needed to be a 'more robust social partnership between patients, practitioners and policy-makers'.[2] Further schemes would be cancelled unless they met local capacity demands and could demonstrate value for money.[3] The private sector was reported to be unsettled by the possibility that the budget for ISTCs could be halved. Delegates at Laing & Buisson's inaugural Independent Healthcare Convention, notably those from Nuffield and Spire Healthcare (which had recently purchased BUPA's portfolio of hospitals), were said to be 'still unsure about the future direction of the NHS'. In his keynote address to the Convention, Nuffield's chief executive David Mobbs said that 'After four years of endless bureaucracy and considerable investment, independent sector providers were starting to wonder if they were wasting their time".[4]

On 15 November, however, a ministerial statement from the Department of Health clarified the situation, at least with regard to Phase 2 contracts.[5] Johnson said that following a 'thorough revalidation of all the schemes currently being procured nationally through the ISTC programme' he had 'accepted the advice of

the Director General of the Commercial Directorate of the DH
to proceed with 10 schemes, 3 of which had been approved to
move to financial close'.* But six schemes would 'not proceed as
they were unlikely to provide acceptable value for money as the
local NHS has successfully improved capacity to meet patients'
needs'.**

Johnson 'reaffirmed the Government's commitment to using a
range of providers to deliver high quality health services'. As well
as confirming that 'independent sector provision beyond the current round of procurements, [would] be procured locally rather
than centrally', the Health Secretary also 'set out details of how
the Department will ensure there is a level playing field for all
NHS providers in future'. These included:

- A new forum for independent sector providers to advise the
  Department on local procurement practice;
- Extending NHS indemnity cover (the Clinical Negligence
  Scheme for Trusts) to non-NHS providers of NHS services;
- Plans to promote patient choice and make patients more
  aware that they can be seen by private sector providers free
  of charge if they choose;
- New guidance to the NHS about how it should work with
  the private and voluntary sector;
- A continuing role for the independent sector in helping to
  improve primary care services and providing additional GP
  surgeries.

*These were: PET CT North Diagnostics (additional CT scans); PET CT South Diagnos-
tics (additional CT scans); Renal (provision of dialysis treatment); Hampshire and Isle
of Wight Electives (Southampton element); Greater Manchester (B) Clinical Assessment
and Treatment Services; Avon, Gloucestershire and Wiltshire Electives; Essex Electives;
Hertfordshire Electives; Greater Manchester (A) Clinical Assessment and Treatment Services; London North Electives.

**The cancelled schemes were: North East Yorkshire and North Lincolnshire Refer-
ral Assessment Diagnostics and Treatment Service; North East Diagnostics; South East
Diagnostics; Norfolk, Suffolk and Cambridge Electives; Cumbria & Lancashire Clinical
Assessment and Treatment Services; Hampshire and Isle of Wight Electives (Lymington
element).

Mr Johnson also told the House of Commons: 'I am today providing further information on each first wave scheme, including the contract value, volume of activity, case mix by volume and utilisation rates, and in future this data will be published annually.'

Several points in these statements call for comment. First, there was to be no 'Phase 3' of the ISTC programme. Johnson had already told the Health Select Committee in July, shortly after taking office, that 'I don't believe there is the need for another independent sector treatment centre (ISTC) procurement and there won't be a third wave'. However the industry journal *HealthInvestor* dismissed this as a case of 'all spin and no substance', adding: 'The DH never seriously considered launching a third wave. Once the remaining projects in the current second wave are signed, and a quasi-market established, all future ISTCs were to be procured by individual primary care trusts.'[6]

Second, it looked at first sight as if Phase 2 of the ISTC programme had been radically reduced. Moreover the most controversial element in the programme, the introduction of CATS, has been limited to two schemes in Greater Manchester. Those planned for the northwest and northeast have gone, with no word of any new ones. On the other hand, as mentioned earlier, the shape of Phase 2 has become distinctly elastic, capable of incorporating a broad range of service models (including CATS, the Extended Choice Network and primary care) that will be attractive to investors, going well beyond the type of fixed site establishment offering a limited range of elective procedures comprised in Wave 1. While the ministerial statement refers to 'a reduction in the overall size of the procurement' [of ISTCs], the total amount of money set aside for Phase 2 is not being reduced.[7] The £4bn. budget is effectively ring-fenced.

What these two policies taken together seem to imply is not a reversal of the drive to move from an integrated national health service to a healthcare market increasingly focused on profitability, but rather a change of focus: a switch from a national to a local programme of procurement of an extended range of services from the private sector, but with the overall scale of funding unchanged, if not expanded. For example, the incoming Director General of the Commercial Directorate, Channing Wheeler, told the Independent Healthcare Convention mentioned above that the Extended Choice Network of private providers would become 'more profound' in future,[8] and that patient choice would in time deliver far greater volumes than those commissioned through the ISTCs.[9] The extension of the Clinical Negligence Scheme for Trusts to all non-NHS providers of NHS care will further normalise the use of for-profit providers within the NHS, and significantly ease the cost of market entry.

It may also be remembered that the DH told the Health Committee that the ECN would offer treatments to NHS patients at the NHS tariff on 'ad hoc basis', but it is now clear that companies will only provide treatments at or near tariff if they are guaranteed a predictable supply of them. [10] The Commercial Director of Spire Healthcare, for example, said: 'We are not bound by the tariff when we are called in as a distress purchase [i.e. a spot purchase] caused by the need to treat patients urgently... It costs us more because we cannot plan our spare capacity in the way we can when patients choose to use us, or the primary care trust has a longer-standing contract. It would be better value for the NHS if we were able to treat NHS patients in a planned way...'[11]

Another straw in the wind was a statement by Sir William Wells, the chair of the Board of the Commercial Directorate which had been 'charged with introducing Independent Sector Providers to the NHS'. [12] Sir William said that the board had decided 'to bring ourselves to an end', as ministers had stopped coming to hear its advice and because a 'change in direction' that had ended central contracts for treatment centres and diagnostics meant it had 'served its useful purpose'.[13] Instead, as Johnson's statement indicates, private providers will now have the role of advising the DH on *local* procurement practice through the creation of an Independent Sector Procurement Forum. This forum will evidently be assisted by a similar shift in emphasis by the Commercial Directorate, which 'is being revamped. It will no longer be a semi-freestanding central purchasing authority, but will be reduced in size and regionalised – becoming a consultancy body to primary care trusts, which are to take over locally the purchasing of independent-sector care for NHS patients'.[14] PCTs will also be able, and if their experience under Wave 1 is any guide, strongly encouraged, to use as their commissioners of care one or more of the fourteen major UK and US insurance companies which have already been lined up to be available through 'call-off' framework agreements.[15]

The recent appearance of large numbers of primary care procedures in the total number of procedures said to have been accomplished 'within the ISTC programme' (see Table 4) points in the same direction – the 'continuing role for the private sector in helping to improve primary care services', referred to in Johnson's statement of 15 November. The health minister Ben Bradshaw told the *Financial Times* in November: 'There will be enormous [private-sector] opportunities in the expansion of primary and community care facilities. That's where people should be turning their attention - and they are. There is a lot of interest in health centres and polyclinics.'[16] It was reported that the government was planning a 'charm offensive to persuade the private sector to bid to run over 250 new family doctor practices and health centres across England', in its drive to 'assure the private sector that there has been no change of policy over it having a bigger role in the provision of National Health Service care, despite a cut in the original plans for independent sector treatment centres'.[17]

To summarise: the original ISTC programme, rationalised in terms of adding capacity to reduce waiting times for elective care, has achieved its most fundamental goals: normalising the use of private companies as providers of NHS secondary care, and forcing the restructuring of the domestic private healthcare industry to be able to compete via the ECN. The next phase will be much more diverse. The 'reconfiguration' of secondary care on the lines advocated in Lord Darzi's reports will see a much greater variety in purchasing from private providers, private provision being locally procured but under central direction – i.e. guided by the

Commercial Directorate, which in turn will be responding to advice from the new advisory forum of independent providers.

If these are reasonable inferences to draw from the government's policy statements, the private sector's role in the NHS, far from being reduced, is set to expand and accelerate; and because it will be locally procured it will be even harder to monitor and hold accountable. The destabilisation of NHS trusts, and the implications for the NHS workforce, remain constants in the effects of the policy. A recent example reported in the *Wimbledon Guardian* deserves to be quoted in full, as a suitable conclusion to these reflections:

> Kingston Hospital's £1.6m plan for a private company to run its elective care is the only way to combat falling numbers of patients, according to the hospital's chief executive Carole Heatly. She said that turning to the private sector was the best way for the hospital to increase the quantity of its elective care - a necessary safeguard against losing its training status. If the 10-year deal is brokered, a private company will take control of the hospital's new surgical centre, day unit and eye unit. It would also be put in charge of the hospital's small private ward, Coombe Wing, which it might be able to extend, with profits shared between the hospital and the private company. It is also hoped that the company would expand the hospital's catchment area, making the most of the patient's power to choose a hospital, by marketing its services to GPs and potential patients. Staff would remain employed by the NHS for at least two years but they would be seconded to the private company, who would manage them. Ms. Heatly said that, after two years, staff may be able to choose to be employed by the private company and that in similar set ups across the country, many staff had chosen this option. Nora Pearce, hospital midwife and Unison representative, said: "The hospital has always said its most valuable asset is the staff. Now what are they doing? Selling their most valuable commodity."[18]

Notes

1   Nicholas Timmins and Ben Hall, 'Policy shift on private surgical centres', *Financial Times*, Jul 05, 2007.

2   Ibid.

3   'Health secretary confirms only 'some' wave two ISTCs will go ahead', *Healthcare Market News*, September 2007.

4   'Convention Report: Providers still unsure about future direction of the NHS', *Healthcare Market News*, October 2007.

5   'Johnson outlines new measures to deliver more choice and faster treatment to patients', Department of Health, 15 November 2007.

6 ' All spin and no substance', *HealthInvestor*, September 2007

7   Telephone conversation with the Commercial Directorate, 24 July 2007.

8   Liz Fox, 'Private sector promised more NHS involvement', *Hospital Doctor*, September 14 2007.

9   Nicholas Timmins, 'Hospital chief casts doubt on NHS links', *FT.com site*, September 12, 2007.

10 Nicholas Timmins, 'Last-minute private ops 'cost NHS more', *Financial Times*, November 15 2007.

11 Ibid.

12 Department of Health: '*Working with the Commercial Directorate – A Guide to Commercial Commissioning*' (2006, p4).

13 Nicholas Timmins, 'NHS business board calls end to "waste of time"', *Financial Times*, September 25, 2007.

14 Nicholas Timmins, 'Advisers hit out on NHS cash, *Financial Times*, December 4 2007.

15 Nicholas Timmins, 'Health trusts keen to sign private deals', *Financial Times*, October 9, 2007.

16 Nicholas Timmins,'Private sector alarmed at cuts to NHS work', *Financial Times*, November 14 2007.

17 Nicholas Timmins, 'Private health centre bids urged', *Financial Times*, December 12 2007.

18 Lisa Williams 'Hospital chief: privatization is the best way forward', *Wimbledon Guardian*, 5 December 2007.

Appendix

Department of Health, Freedom of Information response
DE00000249312, received 22 November 2007.

Dear Mr Player,

Thank you for your email of 30 October to the Department of Health requesting further clarification on the CATS, ICATS, CASS and CATC acronyms in relation to Phase 2 of the independent sector treatment centre (ISTC) programme. I have been asked to reply.

Clinical Assessment, Treatment and Support (CATS) services are a collaborative approach to clinical assessment at a more specialised level than is typically currently available in primary care. The CATS service is designed to introduce services in those specialities which most require additional capacity to meet and sustain the 18 week waiting times target, where a considerable amount of the care pathway can be managed in a primary care setting in line with the recommendations of the January 2006 White Paper, Our Health, Our Care, Our Say. For clarity, there are three proposed CATS schemes for the North West area within Phase 2 of the independent sector programme.

In Greater Manchester the CATS schemes, which form part of the Phase 2 independent sector procurements, were originally called Integrated Clinical Assessment and Treatment Services (ICATS). However, in November 2006, the NHS North West changed this to Clinical Assessment, Treatment and Support Services and confirmed that henceforth the schemes should be known as CATS. This decision was made in order to be consistent with the proposed Cumbria and Lancashire scheme which had always been referred to as CATS.

The Clinical Assessment Service Spoke (CASS) was part of the proposed ISTC Phase 2 London South Elective Scheme. This preferred "Hub and Spoke" model offered the prospect of a service delivery model and comprises elective surgical care centres (the Hubs), together with the support of a number of CASS facilities geographically located for ease of patient transport and access.

The CASS facilities proposed a range of healthcare professionals' outreach outpatient services (the Spokes) through integrated health assessment and treatment that covered a range of specialty services including vertically integrated services, diagnostic testing, pre-admission assessment and outpatient services including pre and postoperative care, physiotherapy and rehabilitation services, and minor treatment rooms.

In response to recommendations raised during the case mix review by the NHS London in January, the proposed service delivery model was revised to reflect the Phase 2 London North Electives scheme preference, and the CASS component was adapted to delivery a CATC model. The London South Phase 2 electives scheme was withdrawn in June.

In full, CATCs are part of the proposed ISTC Phase 2 London North Elective Scheme, designed specifically to satisfy the aspirations of Our Health, Our Care, Our Say by providing a comprehensive range of healthcare services in a local community setting across north London. The proposed model would achieve this through the use of a CATC model, independent of the provision of elective day surgery through Surgical Treatment Centres (STCs).

The CATC model offers integrated health assessment and treatment covering a range of specialty services. The full scope of service delivery includes clinical triage, assessment, first line diagnostics and treatment planning, pre-procedural assessment, minor treatment room procedures, follow up outpatients and integrated therapist-led rehabilitation services.

The CATC model provides a separate facility through which the patient can access services in the local community, whilst also providing a key referral link into the more formal elective setting where appropriate. All of the CATC procedural case mix can be performed in a clean room setting through a "one-stop" service pathway wherever appropriate.

I hope this clarifies the situation for you.